SpringerBriefs in Electrical and Computer Engineering

For further volumes:
http://www.springer.com/series/10059

Aris Gkoulalas-Divanis • Grigorios Loukides

Anonymization of Electronic Medical Records to Support Clinical Analysis

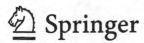

Aris Gkoulalas-Divanis
IBM Research - Ireland
Damastown Industrial Estate
Mulhuddart, Ireland

Grigorios Loukides
Cardiff University
The Parade
Cardiff
United Kingdom

ISSN 2191-8112 ISSN 2191-8120 (electronic)
ISBN 978-1-4614-5667-4 ISBN 978-1-4614-5668-1 (eBook)
DOI 10.1007/978-1-4614-5668-1
Springer New York Heidelberg Dordrecht London

Library of Congress Control Number: 2012948006

Printed on acid-free paper

Springer is part of Springer Science+Business Media (www.springer.com)

Preface

This book grew out of the work of the authors on the problem of preserving the privacy of patient data, which started when they were postdoctoral researchers in the Health Information Privacy Laboratory, Department of Biomedical Informatics, Vanderbilt University. Part of their work was to understand the privacy threats that disseminating clinical data entails and to develop methods to eliminate these threats. The use of data derived from the Electronic Medical Record (EMR) system of the Vanderbilt University Medical Center enabled the authors to realize and appreciate the complexity of the problem and to gain valuable insights that led to developing practical solutions.

The structure of the book closely follows the order in which the authors undertook this research, and some of their works formed the basis of the material presented in this book. We started by realizing that disseminating EMR data requires addressing many important, and often unexplored, privacy issues. One of the main issues was to examine the re-identifiability of diagnosis codes. Towards this goal, we studied a range of attacks that may lead to patient re-identification and performed empirical studies to demonstrate the feasibility of these attacks. Using several large EMR datasets, we showed that the attacks we considered pose a serious privacy threat, which cannot be addressed by popular approaches. The work won a Distinguished Paper Award from the American Medical Informatics Association (AMIA) Annual Symposium in 2009 and appeared in a revised and extended form in the Journal of the American Medical Informatics Association (JAMIA). Having realized the importance of guaranteeing both data privacy and the usefulness of data in biomedical applications, we designed the first approach which guarantees that the disseminated data will be useful in validating Genome-Wide Association Studies. These studies attempt to find clinically meaningful associations between patients' diagnosis and genetic variations, and are considered as the holy grail of personalized medicine. The work was published in the Proceedings of the National Academy of Sciences in 2010 and was reported by the National Human Genome Research Institute (NHGRI) among the important advances in the last 10 years of genomic research (Eric D. Green, et al. in Nature, vol. 470, 2011). We also gained useful insights on the problem and future directions, when we were preparing two tutorials that were presented at the European Conference on Machine Learning and Principles and Practice of Knowledge Discovery in Databases (ECML/PKDD) in 2011, and at the SIAM International Conference on Data Mining (SDM) in 2012. The slides of these tutorials serve as a helpful companion to the book and can be found at http://www.zurich.ibm.com/medical-privacy-tutorial/ and http://www. siam.org/meetings/sdm12/gkoulas_loukides.pdf, respectively.

This book is primarily addressed to computer science researchers and educators, who are interested in data privacy, data mining, and information systems, as well as to industry developers, and we believe that the book will serve as a valuable resource to them. Knowledge of data mining or medical methods and terminology is not a prerequisite, and formalism was kept at a minimum to enable readers with general computer science knowledge to understand the key challenges and solutions in privacy-preserving medical data sharing and to reflect on their relation with practical applications. By discussing a wide spectrum of privacy techniques and providing in-depth coverage of the most relevant ones, the book also aims at attracting data miners with little or no expertise in data privacy. The objective of the book is to inform readers about recent developments in the field of medical data privacy and to highlight promising avenues for academic and industrial research.

Dublin, Ireland   Aris Gkoulalas-Divanis
Cardiff, UK   Grigorios Loukides

Acknowledgements

This work would not have been possible without the support of several people. The authors would like to thank Bradley Malin and Joshua Denny for many useful discussions, as well as Sunny Wang for providing access to the data we used in the case study. We would also like to thank Hariklia Eleftherohorinou, Efi Kokiopoulou, Jianhua Shao and Michail Vlachos for their insightful comments that helped the presentation of this work.

We are also grateful to Hector Nazario, Susan Lagerstrom-Fife, Jennifer Maurer and Melissa Fearon from Springer and to the publication team at SpringerBriefs, for their great support and valuable assistance in the preparation and completion of this work. Their editing suggestions were valuable to improving the organization, readability and appearance of the manuscript.

Part of this research was funded by grant U01HG004603 of the National Human Genome Research Institute (NHGRI), National Institutes of Health. Grigorios Loukides' research is also supported by a Royal Academy of Engineering Research Fellowship.

Contents

1   **Introduction** 1
    1.1   The Need for Sharing Electronic Medical Record Data 1
    1.2   The Threat of Patient Re-identification 2
    1.3   Preventing Patient Re-identification 4
    1.4   Aims and Organization of the Book 6
    References 6

2   **Overview of Patient Data Anonymization** 9
    2.1   Anonymizing Demographics 9
        2.1.1   Anonymization Principles 9
        2.1.2   Anonymization Algorithms 12
    2.2   Anonymizing Diagnosis Codes 14
        2.2.1   Anonymization Principles 15
        2.2.2   Generalization and Suppression Models 18
        2.2.3   Anonymization Algorithms 19
    2.3   Anonymizing Genomic Data 26
    References 27

3   **Re-identification of Clinical Data Through Diagnosis Information** 31
    3.1   Motivation 31
    3.2   Structure of the Datasets Used in the Attack 33
    3.3   Distinguishability Measure and Its Application to EMR Data 33
    3.4   Utility Measures 36
    References 38

4   **Preventing Re-identification While Supporting GWAS** 39
    4.1   Motivation 39
    4.2   Background 40
        4.2.1   Structure of the Data 41
        4.2.2   Privacy and Utility Policies 42
        4.2.3   Anonymization Strategy 43
        4.2.4   Information Loss Measure 44

4.3   Algorithms for Anonymizing Diagnosis Codes   45
      4.3.1   Privacy Policy Extraction..   45
      4.3.2   Utility-Guided Anonymization of CLInical
              Profiles (UGACLIP)   47
      4.3.3   Limitations of UGACLIP and the Clustering-Based
              Anonymizer (CBA)   49
References   52

5   Case Study on Electronic Medical Records Data   55
    5.1   Description of Datasets and Experimental Setup   55
    5.2   The Impact of *Simple Suppression* on Preventing Data
          Linkage and on Data Utility   55
    5.3   Utility of Anonymized Diagnosis Codes..............................   57
          5.3.1   Supporting GWAS Validation   58
          5.3.2   Supporting Clinical Case Count Studies.......................   60
    References   64

6   Conclusions and Open Research Challenges   65
    6.1   Threats Beyond Patient Re-identification   66
    6.2   Complex Data Sharing Scenarios   67
    References   68

Index   71

List of Figures

Fig. 2.1   A classification of heuristic search strategies 13

Fig. 2.2   Summary of generalization models 14

Fig. 2.3   An example of: (a) original dataset, and (b), (c) two anonymized versions of it 15

Fig. 2.4   An example of: (a) original dataset containing public and sensitive items, (b) a $(0.5, 6, 2)$-coherent version of it, and (c) a generalization hierarchy 17

Fig. 2.5   Subpartitions created during the execution of *Partition* 21

Fig. 2.6   An example of (a) complete two-anonymous dataset, created by Partition, and (b) 2^2-anonymous dataset, created by Apriori 21

Fig. 2.7   An example of (a) $(0.5, 2, 2)$-coherent dataset produced by Greedy, (b) SARs used by SuppressControl, (c) intermediate dataset produced by SuppressControl, and (d) 0.5-uncertain dataset produced by SuppressControl 24

Fig. 3.1   An example of: (a) original dataset containing patient names and diagnosis codes, (b) a de-identified sample of this dataset, and (c) a generalized sample of this dataset 32

Fig. 3.2   Percentage of patient records in *VNEC* that are vulnerable to re-identification when data are released in their original form 34

Fig. 3.3   Characteristics of the *VNEC* dataset: (a) frequency of the ICD codes, and (b) number of ICD codes per record 35

Fig. 3.4   The result of replacing 401.0, 401.1, and 493.00, in the dataset of Fig. 3.1a, with $(401.0, 401.1, 493.00)$ 36

Fig. 3.5   The five-digit code 250.02 and its ascendants at
           different levels of the ICD hierarchy 37

Fig. 4.1   Biomedical datasets (fictional) and policies employed
           by the proposed anonymization approach: (a) research
           data, (b) identified EMR data, (c) utility policy
           (d) privacy policy, and (e) a five-anonymization for the
           research data 41
Fig. 4.2   Example of a research dataset... 51
Fig. 4.3   Anonymizing the data of Fig. 4.2 using CBA 51
Fig. 4.4   Anonymized dataset produced by applying CBA [5]
           to the dataset of Fig. 4.2 52

Fig. 5.1   Percentage of patient records in $VNEC$ that are
           vulnerable to re-identification when (a) data are released
           in their original form, and (b) when ICD codes in
           $VNEC$, which are supported by at most $s\%$ of records
           in VP, are suppressed... 56
Fig. 5.2   Data utility after applying simple suppression, as it is
           captured by (a) SL, and (b) RSL....................................... 58
Fig. 5.3   Re-identification risk (shown as a cumulative
           distribution function) of clinical profiles 58
Fig. 5.4   Utility constraint satisfaction at various levels of
           protection for: (a) $VNEC$, and (b) $VNEC_{KC}$ 59
Fig. 5.5   Example of a query that requires counting the number
           of patients diagnosed with a certain set of ICD codes 61
Fig. 5.6   Relative Error (RE) vs. k for the single visit case and for
           (a) $VNEC$, and (b) $VNEC_{KC}$ 62
Fig. 5.7   Relative Error (RE) vs. k for the all-visits case and for
           (a) $VNEC$, and (b) $VNEC_{KC}$ 63
Fig. 5.8   Mean of Relative Error (ARE) vs. k for the single-visits
           case and for (a) $VNEC$, and (b) $VNEC_{KC}$ 63

List of Tables

Table 1.1   An example of: (a) original dataset, and
(b) a de-identified version of it 3

Table 2.1   (a) Original dataset, and (b), (c) two different
four-anonymous versions of it...................................... 10

Table 2.2   Summary of privacy principles for guarding against
sensitive information disclosure...................................... 10

Table 2.3   Summary of existing grouping strategies w.r.t. their objectives 13

Table 2.4   Summary of algorithms for preventing identity
disclosure in transaction data publishing 20

Table 3.1   Description of the $VNEC$ dataset 35

Table 5.1   Description of the datasets used...................................... 56

Table 5.2   (a) Percentage of retained disease information after
applying simple suppression with varying s, and
(b) disease information retained after applying simple
suppression with varying s 57

Table 5.3   Satisfied utility constraints for UGACLIP and ACLIP
when $k = 2$ and for (a) the single-visit case, and
(b) the all-visits case 60

Table 5.4   Satisfied utility constraints for UGACLIP and CBA
for the single-visit case when (a) $k = 5$, and (b) $k = 10$............. 61

List of Algorithms

Algorithm 1   Partition$(\tilde{\mathscr{D}},\mathscr{C},\mathscr{H},k)$ 20

Algorithm 2   Apriori$(\tilde{\mathscr{D}},\mathscr{H},k,m)$ 22

Algorithm 3   Greedy$(\mathscr{D},h,k,p)$ 24

Algorithm 4   SuppressControl$(\mathscr{D},\rho)$ 26

Algorithm 5   PPE$(\mathscr{D},\mathscr{F},k)$ 46

Algorithm 6   UGACLIP$(\mathscr{D},\mathscr{P},\mathscr{U},k)$ 48

Algorithm 7   CBA$(\mathscr{D},\mathscr{P},\mathscr{U},k)$ 50

Chapter 1
Introduction

1.1 The Need for Sharing Electronic Medical Record Data

Electronic Medical Record (EMR) systems are complex systems for managing detailed clinical data, such as registration data (e.g., patient names and phone numbers), demographics, billing information (e.g., diagnosis codes), medication and allergies, and laboratory test results [8, 27]. Different types of data are stored in different subsystems of an EMR system, which are accessed by multiple parties with different roles and responsibilities. For instance, the coding staff in a healthcare organization may access the registration and billing subsystems to obtain a patient's name and diagnosis codes. Modern EMR systems allow large amounts of patient data, which are typically not available in disease registries and claim records, to be stored, updated, and exchanged between healthcare providers [19]. Thus, they are increasingly being adopted. According to the 2010 National Ambulatory Medical Care Survey,[1] for example, EMR systems were adopted by 50 % of office-based physicians, increasing more than 30 % from 2009, and the goal is to utilize an EMR for each US citizen by 2014.

The use of data derived from EMR systems is a promising avenue for improving healthcare, for two main reasons. First, these data can be *exchanged* between physicians to help them better diagnose and treat diseases, while allowing patients to receive better services. Second, EMR data can be *disseminated* for purposes beyond primary care, which range from enabling post-marketing safety evaluation to supporting biomedical research [19]. For example, the dissemination of patient demographics and diagnosis codes allows data recipients to perform large-scale, low-cost statistical analysis (e.g., to study correlations between age and diabetes) and data mining tasks, such as classification (e.g., to predict domestic violence [33]) and clustering (e.g., to control epidemics [39]).

---

[1] National Ambulatory Medical Care Survey (NAMCS). http://www.cdc.gov/nchs/ahcd.htm.

A. Gkoulalas-Divanis and G. Loukides, *Anonymization of Electronic Medical Records to Support Clinical Analysis*, SpringerBriefs in Electrical and Computer Engineering, DOI 10.1007/978-1-4614-5668-1_1, © The Author(s) 2013

Another scenario that gains increasing popularity involves the dissemination of EMR data combined with genomic information [18, 21, 34]. For instance, the Electronic Medical Records and Genomics (eMERGE) network consists of a consortium of medical centers that disseminate such data to perform genome-phenome association studies with clinical phenotypes derived from EMR systems [28]. To allow large-scale, cost-effective biomedical studies and the validation of clinically-relevant findings, the dissemination of EMR data combined with genomic information is strongly encouraged and, at times, required by agencies world-wide [17, 29]. For example, the National Institutes of Health (NIH) in the US has established the Database of Genotype and Phenotype (dbGaP) [26], a biorepository to facilitate the dissemination of patient-specific records from disparate investigators, and it requires data involved in all NIH-funded genome-wide association studies to be deposited into it [29]. Other countries, such as the UK, which created the UK Biobank, have chosen to centralize primary collection of data [31].

1.2   The Threat of Patient Re-identification

While the dissemination of EMR data is greatly beneficial for research purposes, it must be performed in a way that addresses privacy concerns. According to a recent survey by the National Partnership for Women & Families,[2] 59 % of patients believe that the widespread adoption of EMR systems will lead to more personal information being lost or stolen, while 51 % believe that the privacy of health information is not currently sufficiently protected. To address these concerns, one must ensure: (i) *security* – stored data are not lost or accessed by unauthorized users, (ii) *secrecy* – no one is able to eavesdrop the data while they are transmitted between authorized users, and (iii) *anonymity* – private and sensitive information about individuals is not disclosed when data are released. In fact, guaranteeing the anonymity of EMR data before these data are widely disseminated is not only an ethical but also a legal requirement for healthcare providers.

Towards this goal, policies that restrict the sharing of patient-specific genomic data in a personally identifiable form are emerging. In the US, for instance, the Privacy Rule of the Health Insurance Portability and Accountability Act (HIPAA) [40] outlines two policies by which de-identification can be performed: (i) *Safe Harbor*, and (ii) *Expert Determination*. The Safe Harbor policy is a cookbook approach enumerating 18 identifiers (i.e., attributes that uniquely identify patients, such as patient names and phone numbers) that must be removed from patients' records in order for the data to be designated as de-identified. The Expert Determination policy, in contrast, states that health information can be shared, if an expert certifies that the risk an attacker can use the disseminated data to perform re-identification is low.

---

[2]National Partnership for Women & Families, Making IT Meaningful: How Consumers Value and Trust Health IT Survey. http://www.nationalpartnership.org/

Table 1.1 An example of: (a) original dataset, and (b) a de-identified version of it

Name	Age	Diagnoses	DNA sequence	Age	Diagnoses	DNA sequence
Anne	18	a b c d e f	GC...C	18	a b c d e f	GC...C
Greg	22	a b e g	CG...A	22	a b e g	CG...A
Jack	53	a e	GG...T	53	a e	GG...T
Tom	27	b f g	CT...T	27	b f g	CT...T
Mary	50	a b	CC...A	50	a b	CC...A
Jim	66	c f	AC...C	66	c f	AC...C
(a)				(b)		

Privacy policies are in place in other countries, such as in UK [2] and Canada [3], as well as in the EU [1]. At the same time, the NIH specified that data submitted to the dbGaP repository should adhere to data sharing regulations [29].

These policies and regulations focus on the privacy threat of *re-identification* (also referred to as *identity disclosure*), which involves the association of an identified individual with their published information, such as their demographics or DNA sequences. To counter this threat, they require *de-identifying data*, i.e., removing patients' identifiers from the shared data, while modifying the values of demographics (e.g., by replacing the age for patients over 89 with a "greater than 89" value). As an example, consider the table shown in Table 1.1a, which represents a set of patients' records. Each record corresponds to a different patient and contains their name, age, diagnosis codes, and DNA sequence. The result of applying de-identification to the data contained in Table 1.1a is shown in Table 1.1b. Clearly, de-identification is a first line of defence against re-identification, which, otherwise, would be straightforward for an attacker to perform.

However, applying de-identification to EMR data is insufficient to prevent patient re-identification in practice. To demonstrate this, Sweeney [35] linked a claims database containing information of 135 K patients disseminated by the Group Insurance Commission to the voter list of Cambridge, Massachusetts, based on patient demographics, including date of birth, zip code and gender. In that attack, William Weld, a former governor of Massachusetts was re-identified. It was also suggested that more than 87 % of US citizens can be identified as a result of data linkage [35]. Many other re-identification attacks have been reported, a summary of which can be found in [14]. These include attacks in which (i) students re-identified individuals in the Chicago homicide database by linking it with the social security death index, (ii) an expert witness re-identified most of the individuals represented in a neuroblastoma registry, and (iii) a national broadcaster re-identified a patient, who died while taking a drug, by combining the adverse drug event database with public obituaries. To illustrate how re-identification may occur, consider the de-identified patient data that are shown in Table 1.1b. Observe that, if we assume that an attacker can find these patients' names, age values, and diagnosis codes in an external dataset, then by performing a simple join, between the voter list and Table 1.1b, the attacker will be able to uniquely associate patients with their published records.

1.3 Preventing Patient Re-identification

Based on the above, it is easy to realize that better approaches for preventing patient re-identification are required. These approaches would be extremely useful in many real-world scenarios, such as those involving the dissemination of EMR and genomic data to dbGaP, as they can be used to satisfy the Expert Determination policy of HIPAA. However, designing such approaches involves addressing the following significant research challenges:

1. *The knowledge an attacker may exploit to perform re-identification is, generally, unknown to data publishers prior to data dissemination.* For example, each of the aforementioned re-identification incidents involved a different type of external dataset, and re-identification was performed based on different attributes. In the case of EMR data combined with genomic information, healthcare organizations must, in fact, deal with the protection of many different types of EMR data from multiple potential attackers, including "insiders" (e.g., malicious healthcare employees) and "external" attackers (e.g., parties with access to bio-repositories).
2. *The de-identified data need to be transformed prior to their dissemination, but in a way that they remain useful.* This is particularly challenging for the type of data we consider, because the number and complexity of biomedical studies grows rapidly. Consequently, it is difficult for healthcare organizations to predict the type of studies that these data may be used for, after they are deposited into widely accessible biorepositories.
3. *It is computationally infeasible to transform data in a way that maximizes both data privacy and data utility [38].* Thus, methods that enable the transformation of data with a desirable trade-off between these two properties must be considered by healthcare organizations.

In the following, we briefly mention how current research addresses these challenges. Our discussion serves only as an introduction to the problem of anonymizing EMR data, combined with genomic information, that we examine in this book. For detailed analysis of these challenges (in the context of relational data publishing), we refer the reader to an excellent survey by Fung et al. [15].

To deal with the first challenge, healthcare organizations often make assumptions about adversarial background knowledge, which are based on general data properties, the availability of external datasets and/or on data sharing policies [23, 35]. For instance, the percentage of US citizens who are estimated to be re-identifiable, based on a combination of their date of birth, five-digit Zip code, and gender, drops from 87 to 0.04 % when the year of birth, three-digit Zip code, and gender of these individuals are published instead. Thus, a healthcare organization may decide to publish data that contains more coarse information about patients. There is a considerably large body of research on methods that can be used to estimate the re-identification risk [5, 11–14]. However, these methods focus mostly on the publishing of patient demographics. Recently, an interesting approach that makes no assumptions about an attacker's background knowledge was proposed [6, 10].

This approach proposes a privacy principle, called *differential privacy*, which ensures that the outcome of a calculation is insensitive to any particular record in the dataset. Enforcing this principle offers privacy, because the inferences an attacker can make about an individual will be (approximately) independent of whether any individual's record is included in the dataset or not. Unfortunately, the approach of [6, 10] may produce patient data that are not truthful (i.e., data in which patients are associated with false information). Thus, this approach is inapplicable in the setting we consider.

The second and third challenge call for methods to transform data prior to their dissemination, as well as for ways to quantify data utility and privacy protection. Unfortunately, EMR data transformation cannot be performed by methods that employ encryption and access control [9,32,36], as these data must be disseminated beyond a number of authorized users or be publicly released. *Perturbative* methods are not applicable either, because, in order to prevent re-identification, they modify the values of some attributes in a way that they no longer correspond to real individuals. Perturbative methods are based, for example, on noise addition, or attribute-value swapping among records [4,7,30]. Consequently, the data produced by perturbative methods cannot be analyzed at a patient-level. This is, however, crucial for various clinical studies, such as for determining the number of patient records that harbor a specific combination of diagnosis codes, which is important in epidemiology. Therefore, non-perturbative methods, which transform the data in a way that they can still be analyzed at a patient level, are preferred. Non-perturbative methods work by either deleting records or values from the data prior to their dissemination, or by replacing values with more general ones [35,38]. The transformation of data by non-perturbative methods to prevent identity disclosure is referred to as *anonymization*.

As for measuring data utility, there are two general approaches [20], the first of which measures the information loss incurred during data transformation. Assuming that data are transformed by deleting entire records, this approach would express data utility based on the number of records that have been deleted, for example. The second approach for measuring data utility considers the task that the disseminated data are intended for. Then, data utility is expressed based on how well the disseminated data support this task, compared to the original data. As an example, consider that the data shown in Table 1.1b need to be disseminated to support a task, in which the average age of these patients needs to be determined. It is easy to see that the average age of a patient in the original data is 39.3. If these data was anonymized by deleting some records, however, the average age could change. In this case, data utility would be measured, based on how much the average age of the transformed data differs from 39.3. Having quantified data utility, healthcare organizations can balance it with privacy protection by either constraining one of these two properties and attempting to optimize the other one, or by attempting to transform data in a way that directly optimizes the trade-off between data utility and privacy protection [24,25].

1.4   Aims and Organization of the Book

In this book, we study the problem of privacy-preserving dissemination of EMR data, combined with genomic sequences. This is an important, practical problem, as such data are increasingly required to be shared to support biomedical studies, without comprising patient privacy.

To acquaint the reader with the problem and the techniques that have been proposed to solve it, in Chap. 2, we provide a survey of anonymization techniques. We discuss techniques that are designed to protect different types of patient data, including demographics and genomic sequences, and detail the privacy principles, as well as the optimization and algorithmic strategies they employ.

In Chap. 3, we present an attack that can associate patients with their diagnoses and genomic information [22]. The attack involves linking the disseminated data with external, identified datasets, based on diagnosis codes. We discuss the type of datasets that are involved in the attack and study its feasibility in a real data publishing scenario. This scenario involves de-identified patient data that are derived from the EMR system of Vanderbilt University Medical Center [37] and are combined with genomic sequences [34]. Examining the feasibility of the attack in this setting is of great practical importance, as these data are to be submitted to dbGaP.

As it is demonstrated in Chap. 3, the attack poses a serious threat to patient privacy. Thus, in Chap. 4, we examine how EMR data can be published in a way that prevents the attack, while remaining useful for biomedical analysis. We present an overview of a recent approach [16, 23] that works by transforming diagnosis codes that may lead to re-identification, while preserving the associations between sets of diagnosis codes and genomic sequences that are useful in the intended analytic tasks.

Chapter 5 presents a case study using the EMR datasets that were considered in Chap. 2. Specifically, experiments that demonstrate (i) the inability of popular strategies to prevent the attack while retaining data utility, and (ii) the effectiveness of the approach discussed in Chap. 3 in terms of producing data that remain useful for the intended genomic analysis and general biomedical tasks, are presented.

In Chap. 6, we conclude this work by providing guidance as to what further research is needed to preserve the privacy of patient data. In this respect, we discuss threats to patient privacy that are beyond re-identification, as well as alternative EMR data publishing scenarios.

References

1. EU Data Protection Directive 95/46/ECK (1995)
2. UK Data Protection Act (1998)
3. Personal Information Protection and Electronic Documents Act (2000)

4. Adam, N., Worthmann, J.: Security-control methods for statistical databases: a comparative study. ACM Comput. Surv. **21**(4), 515–556 (1989)
5. Benitez, K., Loukides, G., Malin, B.: Beyond safe harbor: automatic discovery of health information de-identification policy alternatives. In: ACM International Health Informatics Symposium, pp. 163–172 (2010)
6. Blum, A., Dwork, C., McSherry, F., Nissim, K.: Practical privacy: the sulq framework. In: PODS, pp. 128–138 (2005)
7. Dalenius, T., Reiss, S.: Data swapping: A technique for disclosure control. Journal of Statistical Planning and Inference **6**, 731–785 (1982)
8. Dean, B., Lam, J., Natoli, J., Butler, Q., Aguilar, D., Nordyke, R.: Use of electronic medical records for health outcomes research: A literature review. Medical Care Reseach and Review **66**(6), 611-638 (2010)
9. Diesburg, S.M., Wang, A.: A survey of confidential data storage and deletion methods. ACM Computing Surveys **43**(1), 1–37 (2010)
10. Dwork, C.: Differential privacy. In: ICALP, pp. 1–12 (2006)
11. Emam, K.E.: Methods for the de-identification of electronic health records for genomic research. Genome Medicine **3**(4), 25 (2011)
12. Emam, K.E., Dankar, F.K.: Protecting privacy using k-anonymity. Journal of the American Medical Informatics Association **15**(5), 627–637 (2008)
13. Emam, K.E., Dankar, F.K., et al.: A globally optimal k-anonymity method for the de-identification of health data. Journal of the American Medical Informatics Association **16**(5), 670–682 (2009)
14. Emam, K.E., Paton, D., Dankar, F., Koru, G.: De-identifying a public use microdata file from the canadian national discharge abstract database. BMC Medical Informatics and Decision Making **11**, 53 (2011)
15. Fung, B.C.M., Wang, K., Chen, R., Yu, P.S.: Privacy-preserving data publishing: A survey on recent developments. ACM Comput. Surv. **42** (2010)
16. Gkoulalas-Divanis, A., Loukides, G.: PCTA: Privacy-constrained Clustering-based Transaction Data Anonymization. In: EDBT PAIS, p. 5 (2011)
17. Guttmacher, A.E., Collins, F.S.: Realizing the promise of genomics in biomedical research. Journal of the American Medical Association **294**(11), 1399–1402 (2005)
18. Kullo, I., Fan, J., Pathak, J., Savova, G., Ali, Z., Chute, C.: Leveraging informatics for genetic studies: use of the electronic medical record to enable a genome-wide association study of peripheral arterial disease. Journal of the American Medical Informatics Association **17**(5), 568–574 (2010)
19. Lau, E., Mowat, F., Kelsh, M., Legg, J., Engel-Nitz, N., Watson, H., Collins, H., Nordyke, R., Whyte, J.: Use of electronic medical records (EMR) for oncology outcomes research: assessing the comparability of EMR information to patient registry and health claims data. Clinical Epidemiology **3**(1), 259–272 (2011)
20. LeFevre, K., DeWitt, D., Ramakrishnan, R.: Mondrian multidimensional k-anonymity. In: ICDE, p. 25 (2006)
21. Lemke, A., Wolf, W., Hebert-Beirne, J., Smith, M.: Public and biobank participant attitudes toward genetic research participation and data sharing. Public Health Genomics **13**(6), 368–377 (2010)
22. Loukides, G., Denny, J., Malin, B.: The disclosure of diagnosis codes can breach research participants' privacy. Journal of the American Medical Informatics Association **17**, 322–327 (2010)
23. Loukides, G., Gkoulalas-Divanis, A., Malin, B.: Anonymization of electronic medical records for validating genome-wide association studies. Proceedings of the National Academy of Sciences **17**(107), 7898–7903 (2010)
24. Loukides, G., Shao, J.: Capturing data usefulness and privacy protection in k-anonymisation. In: SAC, pp. 370–374 (2007)
25. Loukides, G., Shao, J.: Preventing range disclosure in k-anonymised data. Expert Systems with Applications **38**(4), 4559–4574 (2011)

26. Mailman, M., Feolo, M., Jin, Y., Kimura, M., Tryka, K., Bagoutdinov, R., et al.: The ncbi dbgap database of genotypes and phenotypes. Nature Genetics **39**, 1181–1186 (2007)
27. Makoul, G., Curry, R.H., Tang, P.C.: The use of electronic medical records communication patterns in outpatient encounters. Journal of the American Medical Informatics Association **8**(6), 610–615 (2001)
28. McCarty, C.A., et al.: The emerge network: A consortium of biorepositories linked to electronic medical records data for conducting genomic studies. BMC Medical Genomics **4**, 13 (2011)
29. National Institutes of Health: Policy for sharing of data obtained in NIH supported or conducted genome-wide association studies. NOT-OD-07-088. 2007.
30. Nin, J., Herranz, J., Torra, V.: Rethinking rank swapping to decrease disclosure risk. DKE **64**(1), 346–364 (2008)
31. Ollier, W., Sprosen, T., Peakman, T.: UK biobank: from concept to reality. Pharmacogenomics **6**(6), 639–646 (2005)
32. Pinkas, B.: Cryptographic techniques for privacy-preserving data mining. ACM Special Interest Group on Knowledge Discovery and Data Mining Explorations **4**(2), 12–19 (2002)
33. Reis, B.Y., Kohane, I.S., Mandl, K.D.: Longitudinal histories as predictors of future diagnoses of domestic abuse: modelling study. BMJ **339**(9) (2009)
34. Roden, D., Pulley, J., Basford, M., Bernard, G., Clayton, E., Balser, J., Masys, D.: Development of a large scale de-identified dna biobank to enable personalized medicine. Clinical Pharmacology and Therapeutics **84**(3), 362–369 (2008)
35. Samarati, P.: Protecting respondents identities in microdata release. TKDE **13**(9), 1010–1027 (2001)
36. Sandhu, R.S., Coyne, E.J., Feinstein, H.L., Youman, C.E.: Role-based access control models. IEEE Computer **29**(2), 38–47 (1996)
37. Stead, W., Bates, R., Byrd, J., Giuse, D., Miller, R., Shultz, E.: Case study: The vanderbilt university medical center information management architecture (2003)
38. Sweeney, L.: k-anonymity: a model for protecting privacy. IJUFKS **10**, 557–570 (2002)
39. Tildesley, M.J., House, T.A., Bruhn, M., Curry, R., ONeil, M., Allpress, J., Smith, G., Keeling, M.: Impact of spatial clustering on disease transmission and optimal control. Proceedings of the National Academy of Sciences **107**(3), 1041–1046 (2010)
40. U.S. Department of Health and Human Services Office for Civil Rights: HIPAA administrative simplification regulation text (2006)

Chapter 2
Overview of Patient Data Anonymization

2.1 Anonymizing Demographics

2.1.1 Anonymization Principles

Protecting demographics can be achieved using *perturbative* methods, such as noise addition and data swapping [1], as mentioned in the Introduction. However, these methods fail to preserve data truthfulness (e.g., they may change the age of a patient from 50 to 10), which can severely harm the usefulness of the published patient data. *Non-perturbative* methods preserve data truthfulness, and thus are more suitable for anonymizing patient demographics. We will discuss these methods later in this chapter, but, for now, note that they can be used to enforce anonymization principles, such as k-anonymity [17, 18, 58, 59], which is illustrated below.

Definition 2.1 (k-Anonymity). k-Anonymity is satisfied when each tuple in a table $T(a_1, \ldots, a_d)$, where a_i, $i = 1, \ldots, m$ are quasi-identifiers (QIDs), is indistinguishable from at least $k - 1$ other tuples in T w.r.t. the set $\{a_1, \ldots, a_m\}$ of QIDs.

This principle requires each tuple in a table T to contain the same values in the set of quasi-identifier attributes (QIDs) with at least $k - 1$ other tuples in T. Recall from Introduction that the set of quasi-identifiers contains, typically innocuous, attributes that can be used to link external data sources with the published table. Satisfying k-anonymity offers protection against identity disclosure, because the probability of linking an individual to their true record, based on QIDs, is no more than $\frac{1}{k}$. The parameter k controls the level of offered privacy and is set by data publishers, usually to five in the context of patient demographics [17]. We also note that not all attributes in T need to be QIDs (i.e., it may be that $m < d$), and that an individual may not be willing to be associated with some of these attributes. The latter attributes are referred to as *sensitive* attributes (SAs), and we will examine them shortly. The process of enforcing k-anonymity is called k-anonymization, and

A. Gkoulalas-Divanis and G. Loukides, *Anonymization of Electronic Medical Records to Support Clinical Analysis*, SpringerBriefs in Electrical and Computer Engineering, DOI 10.1007/978-1-4614-5668-1_2, © The Author(s) 2013

Table 2.1 (a) Original dataset, and (b), (c) two different four-anonymous versions of it

Id	Postcode	Expense (K)	Id	Postcode	Expense (K)	Id	Postcode	Expense (K)
t_1	NW10	10	t_1	*	10	t_1	NW[10–15]	10
t_2	NW15	10	t_2	*	10	t_2	NW[10–15]	10
t_3	NW12	10	t_3	*	10	t_3	NW[10–15]	10
t_4	NW13	10	t_4	*	10	t_4	NW[10–15]	10
t_5	NW20	20	t_5	*	20	t_5	NW[20–30]	20
t_6	NW30	40	t_6	*	40	t_6	NW[20–30]	40
t_7	NW30	40	t_7	*	40	t_7	NW[20–30]	40
t_8	NW25	30	t_8	*	30	t_8	NW[20–30]	30
(a)			(b)			(c)		

Table 2.2 Summary of privacy principles for guarding against sensitive information disclosure

Reference	Type of sensitive information disclosure
[11, 47, 63, 66, 67]	Value disclosure
[37]	Semantic disclosure
[32, 35, 44, 45, 67]	Range disclosure

it can be performed by partitioning T into groups of at least k tuples, and then transforming the QID values in each group, so that they become indistinguishable from one another. Formally, k-anonymization is explained below.

Definition 2.2 (k-Anonymization). k-Anonymization is the process in which a table $T(a_1, \ldots, a_d)$, where $a_i, i = 1, \ldots, m$ are quasi-identifiers (QIDs), is partitioned into groups $\{g_1, \ldots, g_h\}$ s.t. $|g_j| \geq k$, $j = 1, \ldots, h$, where $|g_j|$ denotes the size of g_j (i.e., number of tuples contained in g_j), and tuples in each g_j are made identical w.r.t. QIDs.

Table 2.1b and c, for example, are both 4-anonymous; *Postcode* is a QID and *Expense* is an SA. These tables were derived by forming two groups of tuples, one containing $\{t_1, \ldots, t_4\}$ and another containing $\{t_5, \ldots, t_8\}$, and then assigning the same value in *Postcode* to all tuples in each group. Specifically, the *Postcode* values in Table 2.1b have been replaced by a value ∗, which is interpreted as "any postcode value", while, in Table 2.1c, by a new value formed by taking the range of all *Postcode* values in a group.

Note that an individual's sensitive information may be disclosed, even when data are anonymized using a "large" k [47]. Specifically, we can distinguish among three types of sensitive information disclosure, which are summarized in Table 2.2. These types of disclosure have not been examined by the medical informatics community, partly because they have not led to reported privacy breaches [16]. However, we report these types of disclosure, for completeness.

Value disclosure involves the inference of an individual's value in a sensitive attribute (SA), such as *Expense* in Table 2.1c. As an example, consider Table 2.1c and an attacker, who knows that an individual lives in an area with *Postcode* = *NW*10. This allows the attacker to infer that this individual's expense is 10 K.

To prevent value disclosure, an anonymization principle, called l-diversity, was proposed in [47]. This principle requires each anonymized group in T to contain at least l "well represented" SA values [47]. The simplest interpretation of "well represented" is "distinct" and leads to a principle called *distinct l-diversity* [37], which requires each anonymized group to contain at least l distinct SA values. Other principles that guard against value disclosure by limiting the number of distinct SA values in an anonymized group are (a,k)-anonymity [66] and p-sensitive-k-anonymity[63]. However, all these principles still allow an attacker to conclude that an individual is likely to have a certain sensitive value, when that value appears much more frequently than others in the group.

A principle, called recursive (c,l)-diversity [47], addresses this limitation, as explained in Definition 2.3.

Definition 2.3 (Recursive (c, l)-diversity). Assume that a table $T(a_1, \ldots, a_m, sa)$, where $\{a_1, \ldots, a_m\}$ are QIDs and sa is an SA, is partitioned into groups $\{g_1, g_2, \ldots, g_h\}$, such that $|g_j| \geq k$, $j = 1, \ldots, h$, and tuples in g_j will have the same values in each QID after anonymization. Given parameters c, l, which are specified by data publishers, a group g_j is (c,l)-diverse when $r_1 < c \times (r_l + r_{l+1} + \ldots + r_n)$, where $r_i, i \in \{1, \ldots, n\}$ is the number of times the i-th frequent SA value appears in g_j, and n is the domain size of g_j. T is (c,l)-diverse when every g_j, $j = 1, \ldots, h$ is (c,l)-diverse.

Recursive (c,l)-diversity requires each group in T to contain a large number of distinct *SA* values, none of which should appear "too" often. Observe, for example, that the second group of Table 2.1c satisfies recursive $(2,2)$-diversity. This is because it contains three distinct values, whose frequencies in descending order are $r_1 = 2, r_2 = 1$ and $r_3 = 1$, and we have $r_1 < 2 \times (r_2 + r_3)$.

More recently, an anonymization principle, called *privacy skyline*, that can prevent attackers with three different types of background knowledge to infer individuals' sensitive values was proposed in [11]. Privacy skyline considers attackers with knowledge about SA values that an individual I does not have, knowledge about SA values belonging to another individual, and knowledge that a group of individuals, in which I is included, has a certain SA value. We believe that this principle is well-suited to achieve protection of datasets that contain familial relationships. However, we do not consider such datasets in this book.

Semantic disclosure occurs when an attacker can make inferences, related to SA values in an anonymous group, that they cannot make by observing the SA values in the entire dataset [37]. Consider, for example, the distribution of *Expense* values in the first group in Table 2.1c, and observe that it differs from the distribution of all values in the same attribute in Table 2.1c. This group risks semantic disclosure, because it reveals information that cannot be inferred from the entire dataset. Semantic disclosure can be thwarted by t-closeness, a principle that calls for limiting the distance between the probability distribution of the SA values in an anonymized group and that of SA values in the whole dataset [37]. The smaller the distance, the higher the level of protection achieved.

Range disclosure occurs when sensitive information is inferred in the form of sensitive values [32, 35, 44, 45, 67]. Consider, for example, that a ten-anonymous group contains three distinct values 10, 11, and 12 K in *Expense*, which is an SA. Knowing that an individual's tuple is contained in this group, an attacker can infer the range (10–12 K) for this individual's expense. Clearly, when this range is "small", the disclosure may be considered as sensitive. Anonymization principles to guard against range disclosure by limiting the maximum range of SA values in a group of tuples have been proposed by Loukides et al. [44] and Koudas et al. [32], while LeFevre et al. [35] proposed limiting the variance of sensitive values instead. Xiao et al. [67] assumed that sensitive ranges are determined by individuals themselves and proposed, *personalized privacy*. This principle forestalls range disclosure by limiting the probability of associating an individual with their specified range, and is enforced through generalizing SA values. This may be inappropriate for medical analysis tasks in which SAs should remain intact. A principle, called *Worst Group Protection* (WGP), which prevents range disclosure and can be enforced without generalization of SA values was proposed in [45]. WGP measures the probability of disclosing any range in the least protected group of a table, and captures the way SA values form ranges in a group, based on their frequency and semantic similarity.

2.1.2 Anonymization Algorithms

Most anonymization algorithms to protect patient demographics work in two steps; first, they form groups of tuples in a way that optimizes data utility and/or privacy protection, and then transform QID values to enforce an anonymization principle. In the following, we review existing algorithms in terms of search strategies, optimization objectives, and value recoding models.

Search strategies Achieving k-anonymization with minimum information loss is an NP-hard problem [4, 8, 49, 68], thus many methods employ heuristic search strategies to form k-anonymous groups. Samarati [58] proposed a binary search on the height of DGHs, LeFevre et al. [33] suggested a search similar in principle to the Apriori [5] used in association rule mining, and Iyengar [31] used a genetic algorithm. Partitioning has also been used to form groups in k-anonymization. LeFevre et al. [34, 35] examined several partitioning strategies including techniques originally proposed for kd-tree construction [22], while Iwuchukwu et al. [30] developed a set of heuristics inspired from R-tree construction [25]. Several k-anonymization algorithms are based on clustering [2, 36, 44, 51, 68]. The main objective of these methods is to form groups that optimize a particular objective criterion. In order to do so, they perform greedy search constructing groups in a bottom-up [2, 36, 44, 51] or a top-down fashion [68]. Figure 2.1 provides a classification of heuristic search strategies according to the type of search they adopt. Furthermore, approximation algorithms for the problem of optimal k-anonymity under (simple) information loss measures have been proposed in [4, 49, 53].

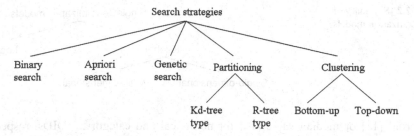

Fig. 2.1 A classification of heuristic search strategies

Table 2.3 Summary of existing grouping strategies w.r.t. their objectives

Reference	Optimization objective	Utility	Sens. inf. protection
[6, 33, 34]	Group-size constrained	Optimal	No guarantee
[8, 35, 68]			
[19]	Utility constrained	Guarantee	No guarantee
[32, 37, 47, 67]	Privacy constrained	Optimal	Guarantee
[44]	Trade-off based	Traded-off with privacy	Traded-off with utility
[46]	Utility-and-privacy constrained	Guarantee	Guarantee

Optimization objectives Anonymization algorithms fall into five categories with respect to their optimization objectives, as can be seen in Table 2.3. *Group-size constrained* algorithms attempt to achieve a maximum level of data utility, subject to a minimum anonymous group size requirement, expressed as k [6, 8, 33–35, 68]. Other algorithms bound the level of information loss incurred during anonymization to ensure that data remain useful for applications, and are referred to as *utility constrained*. However, both group-size and utility constrained algorithms may result in an unacceptably low level of privacy protection from sensitive information disclosure [47]. In response, *privacy constrained* algorithms [32, 37, 47, 67] introduce additional protection constraints (e.g., a minimum level in l-diversity) that released data must satisfy. Another way to deal with utility and privacy is to treat both of them as optimization objectives and attempt to achieve a desired trade-off between them. This *trade-off based* approach, was investigated in [44]. It should be noted, however, that none of the aforementioned approaches can guarantee that data publishers' data utility and privacy protection requirements are satisfied in the anonymized data. In response, a *utility-and-privacy constrained* approach, which allows the specification and enforcement of utility and privacy requirements, was proposed in [46].

Value recoding models After deriving groups of tuples that attempt to optimize their objectives, anonymization algorithms recode QID values using suppression [59], microaggregation [13, 14], or generalization [58, 58]. Suppression suggests eliminating specific QID values, or entire records from the published data [33], while microaggregation involves replacing a group of QID values using the group

Fig. 2.2 Summary of
generalization models

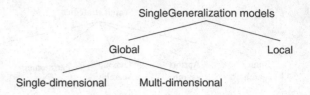

centroid [13] or median value [14] for numerical and categorical QIDs, respectively. Both of these techniques, however, may cause high information loss [33]. Generalization suggests replacing QID values by more general but semantically consistent ones [58, 59]. Thus, suppression can be thought of as the special case of generalization, where all values in a QID are generalized to the most general value (i.e., a value that can be interpreted as any value in the domain of the QID) [4].

Generalization models can be classified into *global* and *local*. Global generalization models involve mapping the domain of QIDs into generalized values [6, 33], and are further grouped into single and multi-dimensional. In the former models, the mapping of a QID value to a generalized value is performed for each QID separately, whereas in the latter ones, the multi-attribute domain of QID values is recoded. On the other hand, in local models, QID values of individual tuples are mapped into generalized values on a group-by-group basis [68]. The different types of generalization models that have been proposed are summarized in Fig. 2.2. For an excellent discussion of these models and formal definitions, we refer the reader to [33, 38].

2.2   Anonymizing Diagnosis Codes

Electronic medical records contain clinical data, such as patients' diagnoses, laboratory results, active medication, and allergies, as discussed in Introduction. While publishing any patient information could, in principle, breach patient privacy, it is important to recognize that publishing different types of information poses different levels of privacy risk. To estimate the level of risk, the principles of *replication* (i.e., the frequency an attribute value appears in an individual's electronic medical record), *resource availability* (i.e., the number and accessibility of datasets, that are external to an individual's electronic medical record and contain the individual's attribute value), and *distinguishability* (i.e., the extent to which one or more attribute values can be used to re-identify an individual) can be used as a guide. These principles build on those defined by the Federal Committee on Statistical Methodology [20] and are acknowledged by health privacy experts [48]. Based on these principles, it can be seen that diagnosis codes have high replication, because an electronic medical record contains all diagnosis codes a patient has been assigned to during multiple hospital visits, and high resource availability, as they are contained in publicly available hospital discharge summaries. Furthermore, as

a Name	Diagnoses
Anne	a b c d e f
Greg	a b e g
Jack	a e
Tom	b f g
Mary	a b
Jim	c f

b Diagnoses
(a,b,c,d,e,f,g)
(a,b,c,d,e,f,g)
(a,b,c,d,e,f,g)
(a,b,c,d,e,f,g)
(a,b,c,d,e,f,g)
(a,b,c,d,e,f,g)

c Diagnoses	
(a,b,c)	(d,e,f)
(a,b,c)	(d,e,f) g
(a,b,c)	(d,e,f)
(a,b,c)	(d,e,f) g
(a,b,c)	
(a,b,c)	(d,e,f)

Fig. 2.3 An example of: (**a**) original dataset, and (**b**), (**c**) two anonymized versions of it

we will explain in the next chapter, diagnosis codes are highly distinguishable. Thus, publishing diagnosis codes may lead to the disclosure of patients' identity [40], and anonymization of diagnosis codes can be employed to eliminate this threat.

2.2.1   Anonymization Principles

Anonymizing diagnosis codes is a challenging computational problem, because only a small number out of thousands of possible diagnosis codes are assigned to a patient. In fact, high-dimensional and sparse data are notoriously difficult to anonymize [3], because, intuitively, it is difficult to find values that are sufficiently similar as to be anonymized with "low" information loss. At the same time, the number of diagnosis codes that are associated to a patient may vary significantly. Due to these reasons, it is difficult to anonymize diagnosis codes by employing the anonymization principles and algorithms that have been designed for demographics and were discussed in Sect. 2.1.1. At the same time, somewhat surprisingly, the medical informatics community has focused on anonymizing demographics [17, 52, 59], but not diagnosis codes. In fact, due to their semantics, a patient-level dataset containing diagnosis codes can be modeled as a transaction dataset. That is, data in which a record (also called *transaction*) corresponds to a different patient and contains the set of diagnosis codes that have been assigned to the patient, as shown in Fig. 2.3a.

To describe transaction data, we employ the terminology of the frequent itemset mining framework [5]. Specifically, diagnosis codes are represented as *items* that are derived from a finite set $\mathscr{I} = \{i_1, \ldots, i_M\}$, such as the set of all ICD-9 codes.[1] A subset I of $\mathscr{I}$ is called an *itemset*, and is represented as the concatenation of the items it contains. An itemset that has m items, or equivalently a *size* of m, is called an m-itemset and its size is denoted with $|I|$. For instance, the set of diagnosis codes $\{a,b,c\}$, in the first record of Fig. 2.3a is a three-itemset. A dataset $\mathscr{D} = \{T_1, \ldots, T_N\}$

---

[1]ICD-9 codes are described in the International Classification of Diseases, Ninth Revision – Clinical Modification, http://www.cdc.gov/nchs/icd/icd9cm.htm

is a set of N records, called *transactions*, and each transaction T_n in $\mathcal{D}$ corresponds to a unique patient. A transaction is a pair $T_n = \langle tid, I \rangle$, where *tid* is a unique identifier,[2] and I is the itemset. A transaction $T_n = \langle tid, J \rangle$ *supports* an itemset I, if $I \subseteq J$. Given an itemset I in $\mathcal{D}$, we use $sup(I, \mathcal{D})$ to represent the number of transactions $T_n \in \mathcal{D}$ that support I. For example, the support of the itemsets $\{a, b\}$ and $\{a, b, c\}$ in the dataset of Fig. 2.3a is 3 and 1, respectively.

Using the above notation, we review anonymization principles for publishing patients' diagnosis codes, starting from the most specific to the more general ones.

Complete k-anonymity A k-anonymity-based principle, called *complete k-anonymity*, for anonymizing transaction datasets was proposed by He et al. [28]. This principle assumes that any itemset (i.e., combination of diagnosis codes) in a transaction can lead to identity disclosure and requires each transaction to be indistinguishable from at least $k - 1$ other transactions, based on any of these combinations. The following definition explains the concept of complete k-anonymity.

Definition 2.4 (Complete k-anonymity). Given a parameter k that is specified by data publishers, a transaction dataset $\mathcal{D}$ satisfies complete k-anonymity when $sup(I_j, \mathcal{D}) \geq k$, for each itemset I_j of a transaction $T_j = \langle tid_j, I_j \rangle$ in $\mathcal{D}$, with $j \in [1, N]$.

Observe that satisfying complete k-anonymity guarantees that an attacker cannot link a patient's identity to fewer than k transactions of the anonymized dataset. For instance, consider the dataset in Fig. 2.3b, in which items a to d have been replaced by a generalized item (a, b, c, d), interpreted as any non-empty subset of $abcd$. This dataset satisfies complete six-anonymity, hence a patient's identity cannot be linked to fewer than six transactions, based on any combination of the diagnosis codes a to d. The authors of complete k-anonymity implicitly assume that attackers may know all the diagnosis codes contained in a patient's transaction. However, this assumption is considered as too strict in most diagnosis code publishing scenarios [41], because, typically, only certain combinations of diagnosis codes of a patient are published [40]. For instance, an attacker who attempts to link the published dataset to hospital discharge records, can only use sets of diagnosis codes that were assigned to a patient during a single hospital visit [40, 41]. Thus, anonymizing a dataset to satisfy complete k-anonymity may result in unnecessary information loss.

k^m-anonymity Terrovitis et al. [60] assume that, due to the semantics of transaction data, it may be difficult for an attacker to learn more than a certain number of a patient's diagnosis codes. Based on this assumption, the authors of [60] proposed k^m-anonymity, which thwarts attackers who know *any* combination of at most m diagnosis codes. This principle is explained in Definition 2.5, and it ensures that no m itemset can be used to associate an individual with fewer than k transactions in the published dataset.

---

[2]The identifier is used only for reference and may be omitted, if this is clear from the context.

a		b	c
Name	*Diagnoses*	*Diagnoses*	(a,b,c,d)
Anne	a b c d e f	(a,b,c,d) e f	
Greg	a b e g	(a,b,c,d) e g	
Jack	a e	(a,b,c,d) e	(a,b) (c,d)
Tom	b f g	(a,b,c,d) f g	
Mary	a b	(a,b,c,d)	
Jim	c f	(a,b,c,d) g	a b c d

Fig. 2.4 An example of: (**a**) original dataset containing public and sensitive items, (**b**) a $(0.5, 6, 2)$-coherent version of it, and (**c**) a generalization hierarchy

Definition 2.5 (k^m-anonymity). Given parameters k and m, which are specified by data publishers, a dataset $\mathscr{D}$ satisfies k^m-anonymity when $sup(I, \mathscr{D}) \geq k$, for each m-itemset I in $\mathscr{D}$.

The dataset shown in Fig. 2.3a, for example, does not satisfy 2^2-anonymity, because the combination of diagnosis codes ac appears only in one transaction. As an example of a dataset that satisfies 2^2-anonymity, consider the dataset shown in Fig. 2.3c. In the latter dataset, items a to c have been replaced by a generalized item (a, b, c), which is interpreted as any non-empty subset of abc, while items d to f have been replaced by (d, e, f). Thus, the dataset of Fig. 2.3c contains at least two transactions that can be associated with any pair of diagnosis codes a to e.

So far, we have discussed how to prevent identity disclosure, which is essential to comply with data sharing regulations [12, 50]. However, ensuring that patients will not be associated with *sensitive* diagnosis codes (i.e., diagnoses that can socially stigmatize patients) is also important. Examples of sensitive diagnosis codes are sexually transmitted diseases and drug abuse, as they are specified in related policies [62]. To see how sensitive information disclosure can be performed, consider Fig. 2.4a, in which the diagnosis codes e to g are sensitive and are denoted with bold letters. An attacker, who knows that a patient is diagnosed with a and b, can associate the patient with the sensitive diagnosis code e with a probability of $\frac{2}{3}$. Clearly, this may not be acceptable when a healthcare provider's policy requires the maximum probability of inferring a patient's sensitive diagnosis to be $\frac{1}{2}$.

Guarding against sensitive information disclosure has been the focus of two recent works in the data management community [43, 69].

(h, k, p)-coherence Xu et al. [69] introduced (h, k, p)-coherence, which treats diagnosis codes that can lead to identity disclosure (i.e., non-sensitive diagnosis codes) similarly to k^m-anonymity and additionally limits the probability of inferring sensitive diagnosis codes using a parameter h. Specifically, the function of parameter p is the same as m in k^m-anonymity, while h is expressed as a percentage. This anonymization principle is explained below.

Definition 2.6 ((h,k,p)-coherence). Given parameters h, k, and p, which are specified by data publishers, a dataset $\mathscr{D}$ satisfies (h,k,p)-coherence when $sup(I,\mathscr{D}) \geq k$, for each p-itemset I comprised of public items in $\mathscr{D}$, and $\frac{sup(I \cup j, \mathscr{D})}{sup(I,\mathscr{D})} \times 100\% \leq h$.

Thus, (h,k,p)-coherence can forestall both identity and sensitive information disclosure. To see this, observe that the dataset in Fig. 2.4b satisfies $(0.5,6,2)$-coherence, and, as such, it prevents an attacker, who knows any pair of diagnosis codes a to d, to infer any of the sensitive codes e to g, with a probability of more than 0.5. This principle assumes that all combinations of p non-sensitive diagnosis codes can lead to identity disclosure and that every diagnosis code needs protection from either identity or sensitive information disclosure. Thus, applying (h,k,p)-coherence in medical data publishing applications, in which only certain diagnosis codes are linkable to external data sources and specific diagnosis codes are sensitive, may unnecessarily incur a large amount of information loss.

ρ-**uncertainty** Another principle to guard against sensitive information disclosure, called ρ-uncertainty, was introduced by Cao et al. [43]. As can be seen from the definition below, ρ-uncertainty limits the probability of associating a patient with any of their sensitive diagnosis codes, using a threshold ρ.

Definition 2.7 (ρ-uncertainty). Given parameter ρ, which is specified by data publishers, a dataset $\mathscr{D}$ satisfies ρ-uncertainty when $\frac{sup(I \cup j, \mathscr{D})}{sup(I,\mathscr{D})} < \rho$, for each I-itemset in $\mathscr{I}$, where j is a sensitive item in $\mathscr{I}$ such that $j \notin I$.

Different from the aforementioned anonymization principles, ρ-uncertainty can be used to thwart attackers who can use any combination of items (either public or sensitive) to infer an individual's sensitive item. Also, due to the monotonicity of support, we have that $sup(I \cup J, \mathscr{D}) \leq sup(I \cup j, \mathscr{D})$, for every J such that $j \subseteq J$. This implies that ρ-uncertainty ensures that any combination of sensitive items that are not known to an attacker will receive protection as well. For instance, the dataset in Fig. 2.4b does not satisfy 0.5-uncertainty, because an attacker, who knows that an individual is associated with $abcd$ and the sensitive item f, can infer that the individual is associated with another sensitive item e with a probability of 0.5. Unfortunately, however, enforcing ρ-uncertainty does not prevent identity disclosure. This implies that this principle is unsuited for being used in scenarios in which preventing identity disclosure is a legal requirement [12, 54, 64], such as those involving the publishing of diagnosis codes.

2.2.2 Generalization and Suppression Models

To enforce the aforementioned anonymization principles, generalization and suppression of items can be applied. The models that have been developed to perform these operations bear some similarity to those that have been proposed for relational uuta [33,38], and they can be classified into *global* and *local* models. *Global* models require generalizing or suppressing all instances (i.e., occurrences) of an item in a transaction dataset in the same way, whereas *local* models do not impose this requirement. The dataset shown in Fig. 2.4b, for example, has been anonymized by applying a global generalization model to the dataset of Fig. 2.4a. Note that all instances of the items a to d have been generalized to (a,b,c,d). While local models are known to reduce information loss, they may lead to the construction of datasets that are difficult to be used in practice. This is because data mining algorithms and analysis tools cannot work effectively on these datasets [23].

A hierarchy-based model, which is similar to the full-subtree generalization model introduced by Iyengar [31] for relational data, was proposed by Terrovitis et al. [60]. This model assumes the existence of a generalization hierarchy, such as the one shown in Fig. 2.4c, and requires entire subtrees of original items (i.e., leaf-level nodes in the hierarchy) to be replaced by a unique internal node in the hierarchy. Consider, for example, the hierarchy in Fig. 2.4c. According to the model proposed in [69], a can be generalized to (a,b) or (a,b,c,d), but not to (a,c), as (a,c) is not represented as an internal node in the hierarchy. This model is not suitable for generalizing diagnosis codes, for two reasons. First, it unnecessarily restricts the number of possible generalizations, which may harm data utility [42]. Second, it is based on hierarchies, which, in the case of diagnosis codes, are either not well-designed (e.g., "too" coarse) or non-existent [56]. He et al. [28] applied the hierarchy-based model in a local manner, allowing different occurrences of the same item to be replaced by different generalized items. In a different line of research, Xu et al. [60] proposed applying global suppression to non-sensitive items, and pointed out that the latter operation has the important benefit of preserving the support of original non-suppressed items. Cao et al. [9] proposed a global suppression model that can be applied to both sensitive and not-sensitive items. Overall, generalization typically incurs a lower amount of information loss than suppression, and global generalization models are preferred due to their ability to preserve data utility in data analysis and mining applications.

2.2.3 Anonymization Algorithms

Similarly to the problem of k-anonymizing demographic data, applying the afore-mentioned principles to anonymize transaction data is NP-hard, when one needs to minimize information loss [42, 60]. Thus, a number of heuristic algorithms have been proposed to deal with this problem, and they can be classified based on the privacy principle they adopt, as illustrated in Table 2.4. In the following, we present these algorithms, reviewing the search and data transformation strategies they adopt.

Partition algorithm He et al. [28] proposed *Partition*, a top-down algorithm to enforce complete k-anonymity. As can be seen in the simplified version of Partition, shown in Algorithm 1, the algorithm gets as input an anonymized dataset $\tilde{\mathcal{D}}$,

Table 2.4 Summary of algorithms for preventing identity disclosure in transaction data publishing

Algorithm	Principle	Search strategy	Transformation
Partition [28]	Complete k-anonymity	Top-down partitioning	Local generalization
Apriori [60]	k^m-anonymity	Bottom-up traversal	Global generalization
LRA [61]	k^m-anonymity	Horizontal partitioning	Local generalization
VPA [61]	k^m-anonymity	Vertical partitioning	Global generalization
Greedy [24]	(h, k, p)-coherence	Greedy search	Global suppression (non-sensitive items)
SuppressControl [42]	ρ-uncertainty	Greedy search	Global suppression (any item)

Algorithm 1   Partition($\tilde{\mathcal{D}}, \mathscr{C}, \mathscr{H}, k$) [28]

---

    input: Dataset $\tilde{\mathcal{D}}$, hierarchy cut $\mathscr{C}$, generalization hierarchy $\mathscr{H}$, parameter k
    output: Complete k-anonymous dataset $\tilde{\mathcal{D}}'$
1.   Start with the most generalized dataset $\tilde{\mathcal{D}}$
2.   **if** complete k-anonymity is not satisfied
3.   **return** $\tilde{\mathcal{D}}$
4.   **else**
5.   Find the node u in $\mathscr{H}$ that incurs minimum information loss when replaced by its immediate ascendants in $\mathscr{H}$
6.   Update $\mathscr{C}$ by replacing u with its immediate ascendants
7.   Update $\tilde{\mathcal{D}}$ based on $\mathscr{C}$
8.   Create subpartitions of $\tilde{\mathcal{D}}'$ such that each of them contains all transactions in $\tilde{\mathcal{D}}'$ that have exactly the same generalized items
9.   Balance the subpartitions so that each of them has at least k transactions
10.   **for each** subpartition $\tilde{\mathcal{D}}''$
11.   Execute *Partition*($\tilde{\mathcal{D}}, \mathscr{C}, \mathscr{H}, k$)

---

a generalization hierarchy $\mathscr{H}$, and a parameter k. $\tilde{\mathcal{D}}$ initially contains a single generalized item that appears in the root of the generalization hierarchy $\mathscr{H}$ and replaces all items. More specifically, $\tilde{\mathcal{D}}$ is constructed based on a hierarchy cut $\mathscr{C}$, i.e., a set of nodes in $\mathscr{H}$, such that every item in the domain $\mathscr{I}$ can be replaced by exactly one node in the set, according to the hierarchy-based generalization model. A hierarchy cut, for example, contains the nodes a, b, and (c, d) in the hierarchy of Fig. 2.4c. The algorithm proposed in [28] works by recursively partitioning $\tilde{\mathcal{D}}$, as long as complete k-anonymity is satisfied. In each execution, Partition is applied to a *subpartition* of at least k transactions in $\tilde{\mathcal{D}}$, which have the same generalized items, and the generalized items in these transactions are replaced by less general ones, in a way that reduces information loss. After Algorithm 1 terminates, all the constructed subpartitions satisfy complete k-anonymity and constitute a partition of the initial anonymized dataset. Thus, these subpartitions are combined into a publishable dataset (this process is straightforward and omitted from Algorithm 1, for clarity).

Partition starts by an anonymized dataset $\tilde{\mathcal{D}}$, in which all items are replaced by the most generalized item (step 1). If $\tilde{\mathcal{D}}$ does not satisfy complete k-anonymity, the

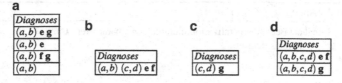

Fig. 2.5 Subpartitions created during the execution of *Partition*

Fig. 2.6 An example of (a) complete two-anonymous dataset, created by Partition, and (b) 2^2-anonymous dataset, created by Apriori

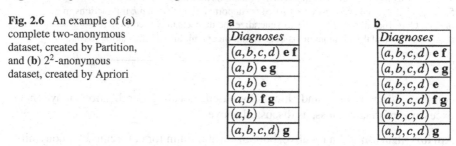

algorithm returns this dataset (steps 2 and 3). Otherwise, it revises the hierarchy cut $\mathscr{C}$ that corresponds to $\tilde{\mathscr{D}}$, by replacing a single node u in $\mathscr{H}$ (the one whose replacement incurs minimum information loss) with its immediate ascendants (steps 5 and 6). After that, Partition updates the transactions in $\tilde{\mathscr{D}}$, so that their generalized items are all contained in the updated hierarchy cut (step 7). This process creates a number of transactions in $\tilde{\mathscr{D}}$ that contain exactly the same generalized items with others. These transactions are identified by the Partition algorithm, which adds them into a subpartition (step 8). Subsequently, the resultant subpartitions are balanced, so that they contain at least k transactions (step 9). This involves redistributing transactions from subpartitions that have more than k transactions to others with fewer than k transactions, and potentially further generalization. Last, Partition is executed using each of these subpartitions as input (steps 10 and 11).

For example, consider applying Partition to anonymize the dataset in Fig. 2.4a, using $k = 2$, and assume that only non-sensitive items are generalized, based on the hierarchy shown in Fig. 2.4c. Initially, Partition is applied to a dataset $\tilde{\mathscr{D}}$ in which all transactions have the most general item (a, b, c, d), and the hierarchy cut contains only (a, b, c, d). The dataset $\tilde{\mathscr{D}}$ satisfies complete three-anonymity, and Parition replaces (a, b, c, d) with (a, b) and (c, d). This results in the three subpartitions, shown in Fig. 2.5a–c. Since the last two subpartitions contain fewer than k transactions, they are merged into the subpartition shown in Fig. 2.5d. Then, the algorithm is executed recursively, first for the subpartition of Fig. 2.5a and then for that of Fig. 2.5d. However, splitting any of these subpartitions further would violate complete two-anonymity, so the algorithm stops. The complete two-anonymous dataset in Fig. 2.6a, which is constructed by combining the subpartitions, can thus be safely released.

The Partition algorithm is efficient and effective for enforcing complete k-anonymity [28]. However, it is not particularly suited for anonymizing diagnosis codes with "low" information loss. This is because, in this setting, applying

Algorithm 2 Apriori($\tilde{\mathscr{D}}, \mathscr{H}, k, m$) [60]

---

    input: Original dataset $\mathscr{D}$, generalization hierarchy $\mathscr{H}$, parameters k and m
    output: k^m-anonymous dataset $\tilde{\mathscr{D}}$
1. $\tilde{\mathscr{D}} \leftarrow \mathscr{D}$
2.   **for** $j = 1$ to m
3.   **for each** transaction T in $\mathscr{D}$
4.   Consider all the j-itemsets of T (generalized or not)
5.   S $\leftarrow$ Find every j-itemset I that is supported by fewer than k transactions in $\mathscr{D}$
6.   Construct all possible ways to generalize the itemsets in S according to $\mathscr{H}$
8. $\tilde{\mathscr{D}}' \leftarrow$ find the k^j-anonymous dataset that incurs minimum information loss
9.   **return** $\tilde{\mathscr{D}}$

---

complete k-anonymity and hierarchy-based, local generalization may incur excessive information loss, as discussed above.

Apriori algorithm An iterative, bottom-up algorithm for enforcing k^m-anonymity, called *Apriori*, was proposed by Terrovitis et al. [60]. Since any superset of an itemset I has a support that is at most equal to that of I, it is possible for itemsets that need protection to be examined in a progressive fashion; from single items to m itemsets. Thus, Apriori generalizes larger itemsets, based on the way their subsets have been generalized [60]. Generalization is performed by traversing the hierarchy in a bottom-up, breadth-first way, using the hierarchy-based, global generalization model that was discussed above. The replacement of the items in an itemset with more general items (i.e., those in the upper levels of $\mathscr{H}$) can increase its support. This helps the enforcement of k^m-anonymity, but increases the level of information loss. Thus, Apriori starts from leaf-level nodes in the hierarchy and then examines the immediate ascendants of these items, one at a time. This is reminiscent to the strategy followed by the Apriori association rule algorithm [5].

An overview of Apriori is provided in Algorithm 2. The algorithm starts with the original dataset $\mathscr{D}$, which is assigned to $\tilde{\mathscr{D}}$, and performs m iterations (steps 1 and 2). In the j-th iteration, it identifies all possible j-itemsets that are not protected in $\tilde{\mathscr{D}}$ and then constructs a k^j-anonymous version $\tilde{\mathscr{D}}$ of $\mathscr{D}$ that incurs minimum information loss (steps 3–8). This is achieved with the use of a data structure, which stores the non-protected itemsets and their generalized counterparts and allows efficient itemset retrieval and support counting [60]. Subsequently, Apriori proceeds into the next iteration, and, after m iterations, it returns a k^m-anonymous dataset (step 10).

To exemplify, we discuss how Apriori can be applied to the dataset shown in Fig. 2.4a to enforce 2^2-anonymity (assume that only non-sensitive items are generalized). Given the hierarchy of Fig. 2.4c, Apriori considers original items first, but the dataset in Fig. 2.4a violates 2^2-anonymity. Thus, the algorithm attempts the generalization of a and b to (a,b) and that of c and d to (c,d). However, neither of these generalizations suffice to protect privacy, and Apriori eventually generalizes all non-sensitive items to (a,b,c,d). The resultant dataset, shown in Fig. 2.6b, is 2^2-anonymous and can be safely published.

LRA and VPA algorithms Terrovitis et al. [61] also proposed two efficient algorithms that are based on Apriori. The first of these algorithms, called *Local Recoding Anonymization* (LRA), splits $\mathscr{D}$ horizontally, so that the transactions in each subpartition share a large number of items and have a similar number of m-itemsets. Specifically, the transactions in $\mathscr{D}$ are sorted based on Gray ordering [26] and then grouped into subpartitions of approximately equal size. This strategy brings together transactions that will incur "low" information loss when anonymized. After that, a k^m-anonymous dataset is constructed by applying Apriori with the same k and m values, in each subpartition separately. LRA scales better with the size of dataset than Apriori, but still much time is spent to anonymize subpartitions that contain large transactions.

To address this issue and further improve efficiency, the authors of [61] proposed *Vertical Partitioning Algorithm* (VPA), which applies hierarchy-based, global generalization and works in two phases. In the first phase, the domain of items $\mathscr{I}$ is split into subpartitions $\mathscr{I}_1, \ldots, \mathscr{I}_l$ that contain items whose common ancestor lies at a certain level in the hierarchy. For example, partitioning together items whose common ancestor lies at the second level of the hierarchy that is shown in Fig. 2.4c, yields the subpartitions (a, b) and (c, d). This process creates a number of datasets $\mathscr{D}_1, \ldots, \mathscr{D}_l$, each containing one subpartition of $\mathscr{I}$. Then, Apriori is applied with the same k and m values to each of the latter datasets. However, the entire dataset may not be k^m-anonymous, if there are item combinations that span multiple subpartitions of $\mathscr{I}$. Thus, in the second phase, VPA constructs a k^m-anonymous dataset by applying Apriori in the dataset that contains all generalized items created during the previous phase.

LRA and VPA are significantly faster than Apriori and achieve a comparable result in terms of information loss [61]. However, they enforce k^m-anonymity, using hierarchy-based generalization, which makes them unsuited for being applied to anonymize diagnosis codes, as mentioned in Sects. 2.2.1 and 2.2.2, respectively.

We now review two suppression-based algorithms, which provide protection from sensitive information disclosure.

Greedy algorithm Xu et al. [69] proposed Greedy, an algorithm that employs suppression to enforce (h, k, p)-coherence. Central to this algorithm is the notion of *mole*, which is defined below.

Definition 2.8 (Mole). Given an original dataset $\mathscr{D}$, and values for the parameters h, k, and p, a *mole* is defined as an itemset I, comprised of public items in $\mathscr{I}$, such that $sup(I, \mathscr{D}) < k$ and $\frac{sup(I \cup j, \mathscr{D})}{sup(I, \mathscr{D})} > h$, for each sensitive item j in $\mathscr{I}$.

Clearly, no (h, k, p)-coherent dataset contains a mole, and item suppression helps the elimination of moles. At the same time, suppression incurs information loss, which needs to be kept at a minimum to preserve the utility of the published data. Thus, Greedy works by iteratively removing public items from a dataset, until the resultant dataset satisfies (h, k, p)-coherence.

As can be seen in the simplified version of Greedy that is presented in Algorithm 3, this algorithm starts by assigning $\mathscr{D}$ to a dataset $\tilde{\mathscr{D}}$ and then suppresses

---

Algorithm 3   Greedy($\mathscr{D}, h, k, p$) [69]

---

    input: Original dataset $\mathscr{D}$, parameters h, k, and p
    output: (h, k, p)-coherent dataset $\tilde{\mathscr{D}}$
1. $\tilde{\mathscr{D}} \leftarrow \mathscr{D}$
2.   **for each** 1-itemset I in $\tilde{\mathscr{D}}$ that is a mole
2. $\tilde{\mathscr{D}} \leftarrow \tilde{\mathscr{D}} \setminus I$
3.   **while** there exists a mole I in $\tilde{\mathscr{D}}$
4.   **for each** public item i in $\tilde{\mathscr{D}}$
5. $MM(i) \leftarrow$ the number of moles in $\tilde{\mathscr{D}}$ that contain item i
6. $IL(i) \leftarrow$ information loss of i
7.   find public item i in $\mathscr{I}$ with the maximum $\frac{MM(i)}{IL(i)}$
8.   suppress i from all transactions in $\tilde{\mathscr{D}}$
9.   **return** $\tilde{\mathscr{D}}$

---

a

Diagnoses
a b e f
a b e g
a e
b f g
a b
g

b

Sensitive Association Rules		
$a \to e$	$a \to f$	$a \to g$
$b \to e$	$b \to f$	$b \to g$
$c \to e$	$c \to f$	$d \to e$
$d \to f$	$e \to f$	$e \to g$
$f \to g$	$f \to e$	$g \to e$
$g \to f$		

c

Diagnoses
a b c d
a b g
a
b g
a b
c

d

Diagnoses
a c d
a g
a
g
a
c

Fig. 2.7 An example of (**a**) $(0.5, 2, 2)$-coherent dataset produced by Greedy [69], (**b**) SARs used by SuppressControl [9], (**c**) intermediate dataset produced by SuppressControl [9], and (**d**) 0.5-uncertain dataset produced by SuppressControl

all moles of size 1 from $\tilde{\mathscr{D}}$ (steps 1 and 2). Next, Greedy iterates over all public items in $\tilde{\mathscr{D}}$, and suppresses the item i with the largest ratio between $MM(i)$, the number of items that contain i, and $IL(i)$, the amount of information loss that suppressing i incurs (steps 3–8). Finding i is performed efficiently using a data structure that organizes moles similarly to the way frequent itemsets are stored in an FP-tree [27]. As for the score IL for an item, it is either determined by data publishers, or set to $sup(i, \mathscr{D})$. The process of suppressing items ends when $\tilde{\mathscr{D}}$ satisfies (h, k, p)-coherence, and, after that, Greedy returns $\tilde{\mathscr{D}}$ (step 9).

To see how Greedy works, consider applying it to the dataset of Fig. 2.4a using $h = 0.5$, $k = 2$, and $p = 2$, when $IL = sup(i, \mathscr{D})$, for each of the public items a to d. The algorithm starts by suppressing d, as it is supported by a single transaction. Then, it suppresses c, because $\frac{MM(c)}{IL(c)} = \frac{3}{2}$ is larger than the corresponding fractions of as all other public items. This suffices to satisfy $(0.5, 2, 2)$-coherence, hence Greedy returns the dataset shown in Fig. 2.7a.

However, Greedy may incur significant information loss if applied to protect diagnosis codes for two reasons. First, it employs (h, k, p)-coherence, which does not take into account detailed privacy requirements that are common in medical data publishing (see Sect. 2.2.1). Second, Greedy uses suppression, which is a rather drastic operation compared to generalization. For instance, enforcing $(0.5, 6, 2)$-coherence using Greedy requires suppressing all public items. On the other hand, there are generalized datasets, such as the one in Fig. 2.4b, that satisfy $(0.5, 6, 2)$-coherence, while incurring much lower information loss.

SuppressControl algorithm Cao et al. [9] have proposed *SuppressControl*, a greedy, suppression-based algorithm to enforce ρ-uncertainty. Central to this algorithm is the notion of *Sensitive Association Rule* (SAR) that is defined below.

Definition 2.9 (Sensitive Association Rule (SAR)). Given an original dataset $\mathscr{D}$, and a value for the parameters ρ, a *sensitive association rule* is defined as an implication $I \rightarrow j$, where I is an itemset in $\mathscr{I}$, called the *antecedent* of $I \rightarrow j$, and j is a sensitive item in $\mathscr{I}$ such that $j \notin I$, called the *consequent* of $I \rightarrow j$.

Given a dataset $\mathscr{D}$ and a set of SARs, the dataset satisfies ρ-uncertainty when, for every SAR $I \rightarrow j$, we have $\frac{sup(I \cup j, \mathscr{D})}{sup(I, \mathscr{D})} \leq \rho$, as can be seen from Definition 2.7. Thus, SuppressControl considers each SAR that can be constructed from the items in $\mathscr{D}$ and suppresses one or more items in the SAR, from all transactions in the latter dataset, until $\mathscr{D}$ satisfies ρ-uncertainty.

Specifically, the algorithm works iteratively, as follows. In the i-th iteration, it finds a set of SARs S whose antecedents contain exactly i items. If such a set cannot be constructed, SuppressControl returns $\tilde{\mathscr{D}}$ (steps 1–5). Otherwise, it updates S by discarding every SAR that does not violate ρ-uncertainty (steps 6 and 7). Next, SuppressControl iterates over all SARs in S, and suppresses items in them, starting with the item l that has the maximum ratio between the number of SARs that contain l and $sup(l, \tilde{\mathscr{D}})$ (steps 9–12). After suppressing l, SuppressControl updates $\mathscr{S}$ by removing all SARs that contain this item (steps 13 and 14), and proceeds into considering the next SAR in $\mathscr{S}$, if there is one. Otherwise, the algorithm proceeds to the next iteration, in which SARs with antecedents larger by one item than those of the SARs considered before, are examined. Last, when all SARs that need protection have been considered, SuppressControl returns $\tilde{\mathscr{D}}$, which satisfies ρ-uncertainty (step 15).

As an example, consider applying SuppressControl to the dataset of Fig. 2.4a, using $\rho = 0.5$. The algorithm starts by constructing all the antecedents of SARs that are comprised of 1 item in this dataset (i.e, a to $\mathbf{g}$), and then discards the SARs that do not need protection, which are highlighted in Fig. 2.7c (steps 1–7). Then, SuppressControl computes the ratios between the NI and support scores for all items, and suppresses the sensitive item $\mathbf{f}$, which has the maximum ratio $\frac{NI(\mathbf{f})}{sup(\mathbf{f}, \mathscr{D})} = \frac{6}{3} = 2$. In this case, the corresponding ratio for $\mathbf{f}$ is also 2, and SuppressControl breaks the tie arbitrarily. Next, the algorithm updates the set of SARs $\mathscr{S}$ by discarding the SARs that contain $\mathbf{f}$ in Fig. 2.7b. After that, the algorithm suppresses the item $\mathbf{e}$ and discards the SARs that contain this item in Fig. 2.7b. At this point, $\tilde{\mathscr{D}}$ is as shown in Fig. 2.7c, and S is empty. Thus, SuppressControl proceeds into the next iteration, in which SAR considers $ab \rightarrow \mathbf{g}$, the only SAR that contains two items in its antecedent and can be formed, based on $\tilde{\mathscr{D}}$. To protect this SAR, the algorithm suppresses b and returns the dataset in Fig. 2.7d, which satisfies 0.5-uncertainty.

Algorithm 4 SuppressControl($\mathscr{D}, \rho$) [9]

    input: Original dataset $\mathscr{D}$, parameter ρ
    output: Dataset $\tilde{\mathscr{D}}$ that satisfies ρ uncertainty
1. $\tilde{\mathscr{D}} \leftarrow \mathscr{D}$
2.   **for each** i from 1 to $|\mathscr{I}|$
3.   S $\leftarrow$ the antecedents of all SARs that contain i items
4.   **if** S $= \varnothing$
5.   **return** $\tilde{\mathscr{D}}$
6.   **for each** SAR $I \rightarrow j$ such that $\frac{sup(I \cup j, \tilde{\mathscr{D}})}{sup(I, \mathscr{D})} \leq \rho$
7.   S $\leftarrow$ S $\setminus \{I \rightarrow j\}$
8.   **while** S $\neq \varnothing$
9.   **for each** item l contained in an SAR in S
10. $NI(l) \leftarrow$ the number of SARs in S that contain item i
11.   find the item l with the maximum $\frac{NI(l)}{sup(l, \tilde{\mathscr{D}})}$
12.   suppress l from all transactions in $\tilde{\mathscr{D}}$
13.   S$_l \leftarrow$ find all SARs in S that contain the item l
14.   S $\leftarrow$ S $\setminus$ S$_l$
15. **return** $\tilde{\mathscr{D}}$

2.3 Anonymizing Genomic Data

While de-identification and anonymization of demographics and diagnosis codes guard against linkage attacks, an individual's record may be distinguishable with respect to genomic data [48]. Lin et al. [39], for example, estimated that an individual is unique with respect to approximately 100 single nucleotide polymorphisms (SNPs), i.e., DNA sequence variations occurring when a single nucleotide in the genome differs between paired chromosomes in an individual. Meanwhile, genomic sequences contain potentially sensitive information, including the ancestral origin of an individual [55] or genetic information about their family members [10], which are likely to be abused, if linked to an individual's identity [57]. To prevent such inferences, only aggregate statistics related to individuals' genetic information were deposited into the public section of dbGaP repository.

    However, Homer et al. [29] have shown that such aggregate statistics may still allow an attacker to infer whether an identified individual belongs to the case or control group of a Genome-Wide Association Study (GWAS) (i.e., if the individual is diagnosed with a GWAS-related disease or not). To achieve this, an attacker needs access to an individual's DNA and to a reference pool of DNA from individuals of the same genetic population as the identified individual (e.g., the publicly available data from the HapMap project.[3]) This allows the attacker to compare the identified individual's SNP profile against the Minor Allele Frequencies (MAFs) [4] of the DNA

---

[3]http://hapmap.ncbi.nlm.nih.gov/
[4]Minor Allele Frequencies (MAFs) are the frequencies at which the less common allele occurs in a given population.

mixture (e.g., the case group in a GWAS) and the reference population, and then to statistically assess the presence of the individual in the "mixture".

The NIH and Wellcome Trust responded to the findings of Homer et al. quickly, by removing genomic summaries of case and control cohorts from the public section of databanks, such as dbGaP [70], while further research investigated the feasibility of Homer's attack [7, 65, 71]. Wang et al. [65] noted that attackers may not have access to MAFs (e.g., when other test statistics are published instead) or to large numbers of independent SNPs from the identified individual and their corresponding allele frequencies from the mixture, which are required for Homer's attack to succeed. Furthermore, Brown et al. [7] showed that many individuals can be wrongly identified as belonging to the case group, because the assumptions about adversarial knowledge made in [29] may not hold in practice. Wang et al. [65] introduced two other attacks that are applicable to aggregate statistics [65]; one that can statistically determine the presence of an individual in the case group, based upon the r^2 measure of the correlation between alleles, and another that allows the inference of the SNP sequences of many individuals that are present in the GWAS data, based on correlations between SNPs.

Recently, Fienberg et al. [21] examined how aggregated genomic data may be published without compromising individuals' privacy, based on *differential privacy* [15]. The latter principle requires computations to be insensitive to changes in any particular individual's data and can be used to provide privacy, as mentioned in Introduction. This is because, differentially private data do not allow an attacker to make inferences about an identified individual that they could not make if the individual's record was absent from the original dataset. In [21], two methods for releasing aggregate statistics for GWAS in a differentially private way were proposed. The first method focuses on the publication of the χ^2 statistic and p-values and works by adding Laplace noise to the original statistics, while the second method allows releasing noisy versions of these statistics for the most relevant SNPs.

References

1. Adam, N., Worthmann, J.: Security-control methods for statistical databases: a comparative study. ACM Comput. Surv. **21**(4), 515–556 (1989)
2. Aggarwal, C., Yu, P.: A condensation approach to privacy preserving data mining. In: EDBT, pp. 183–199 (2004)
3. Aggarwal, C.C.: On k-anonymity and the curse of dimensionality. In: VLDB, pp. 901–909 (2005)
4. Aggarwal, G., Kenthapadi, F., Motwani, K., Panigrahy, R., Zhu, D.T.A.: Approximation algorithms for k-anonymity. Journal of Privacy Technology (2005)
5. Agrawal, R., Srikant, R.: Fast algorithms for mining association rules in large databases. In: VLDB, pp. 487–499 (1994)
6. Bayardo, R., Agrawal, R.: Data privacy through optimal k-anonymization. In: 21st ICDE, pp. 217–228 (2005)
7. Braun, R., Rowe, W., Schaefer, C., Zhang, J., Buetow, K.: Needles in the haystack: identifying individuals present in pooled genomic data. PLoS Genetocs **5**(10), e1000,668 (2009)

8. Byun, J., Kamra, A., Bertino, E., Li, N.: Efficient k-anonymity using clustering technique. In: DASFAA, pp. 188–200 (2007)
9. Cao, J., Karras, P., Kalnis, P., Tan, K.L.: Sabre: a sensitive attribute bucketization and redistribution framework for t-closeness. VLDBJ **20**, 59–81 (2011)
10. Cassa, C., Schmidt, B., Kohane, I., Mandl, K.D.: My sister's keeper? genomic research and the identifiability of siblings. BMC Medical Genomics **1**, 32 (2008)
11. Chen, B., Ramakrishnan, R., LeFevre, K.: Privacy skyline: Privacy with multidimensional adversarial knowledge. In: VLDB, pp. 770–781 (2007)
12. Medical Research Council: MRC data sharing and preservation initiative policy. http://www. mrc.ac.uk/ourresearch/ethicsresearchguidance/datasharinginitiative (2006)
13. Domingo-Ferrer, J., Mateo-Sanz, J.M.: Practical data-oriented microaggregation for statistical disclosure control. IEEE Trans. on Knowledge and Data Engineering **14**(1), 189–201 (2002)
14. Domingo-Ferrer, J., Torra, V.: Ordinal, continuous and heterogeneous k-anonymity through microaggregation. DMKD **11**(2), 195–212 (2005)
15. Dwork, C.: Differential privacy. In: ICALP, pp. 1–12 (2006)
16. Emam, K.E.: Methods for the de-identification of electronic health records for genomic research. Genome Medicine **3**(4), 25 (2011)
17. Emam, K.E., Dankar, F.K.: Protecting privacy using k-anonymity. Journal of the American Medical Informatics Association **15**(5), 627–637 (2008)
18. Emam, K.E., Dankar, F.K., et al.: A globally optimal k-anonymity method for the de-identification of health data. Journal of the American Medical Informatics Association **16**(5), 670–682 (2009)
19. Farkas, C., Jajodia, S.: The inference problem: a survey. SIGKDD Explorations **4**(2), 6–11 (2002)
20. Federal Committee on Statistical Methodology: Report on statistical disclosure limitation methodology. http://www.fcsm.gov/working-papers/totalreport.pdf (2005)
21. Fienberg, S.E., Slavkovic, A., Uhler, C.: Privacy preserving gwas data sharing. In: IEEE ICDM Worksops, pp. 628–635 (2011)
22. Friedman, J., Bentley, J., Finkel, R.: An algorithm for finding best matches in logarithmic time. ACM Trans. on Mathematical Software **3**(3) (1977)
23. Fung, B.C.M., Wang, K., Chen, R., Yu, P.S.: Privacy-preserving data publishing: A survey on recent developments. ACM Comput. Surv. **42** (2010)
24. Gkoulalas-Divanis, A., Loukides, G.: PCTA: Privacy-constrained Clustering-based Transaction Data Anonymization. In: EDBT PAIS, p. 5 (2011)
25. Guttman, A.: R-trees: A dynamic index structure for spatial searching. In: SIGMOD '84, pp. 47–57 (1984)
26. Hamming, R.W.: Coding and Information Theory. Prentice-Hall (1980)
27. Han, J., Pei, J., Yin, Y.: Mining frequent patterns without candidate generation. In: SIGMOD, pp. 1–12 (2000)
28. He, Y., Naughton, J.F.: Anonymization of set-valued data via top-down, local generalization. PVLDB **2**(1), 934–945 (2009)
29. Homer, N., Szelinger, S., Redman, M., et al.: Resolving individuals contributing trace amounts of dna to highly complex mixtures using high-density snp genotyping microarrays. PLoS Genetics **4**(8), e1000,167 (2008)
30. Iwuchukwu, T., Naughton, J.F.: K-anonymization as spatial indexing: Toward scalable and incremental anonymization. In: VLDB, pp. 746–757 (2007)
31. Iyengar, V.S.: Transforming data to satisfy privacy constraints. In: KDD, pp. 279–288 (2002)
32. Koudas, N., Zhang, Q., Srivastava, D., Yu, T.: Aggregate query answering on anonymized tables. In: ICDE '07, pp. 116–125 (2007)
33. LeFevre, K., DeWitt, D., Ramakrishnan, R.: Incognito: efficient full-domain k-anonymity. In: SIGMOD, pp. 49–60 (2005)
34. LeFevre, K., DeWitt, D., Ramakrishnan, R.: Mondrian multidimensional k-anonymity. In: ICDE, p. 25 (2006)

35. LeFevre, K., DeWitt, D., Ramakrishnan, R.: Workload-aware anonymization. In: KDD, pp. 277–286 (2006)
36. Li, J., Wong, R., Fu, A., Pei, J.: Achieving -anonymity by clustering in attribute hierarchical structures. In: DaWaK, pp. 405–416 (2006)
37. Li, N., Li, T., Venkatasubramanian, S.: t-closeness: Privacy beyond k-anonymity and l-diversity. In: ICDE, pp. 106–115 (2007)
38. Li, T., Li, N.: Towards optimal k-anonymization. DKE **65**, 22–39 (2008)
39. Lin, Z., Altman, R.B., Owen, A.: Confidentiality in genome research. Science **313**(5786), 441–442 (2006)
40. Loukides, G., Denny, J., Malin, B.: The disclosure of diagnosis codes can breach research participants' privacy. Journal of the American Medical Informatics Association **17**, 322–327 (2010)
41. Loukides, G., Gkoulalas-Divanis, A., Malin, B.: Anonymization of electronic medical records for validating genome-wide association studies. Proceedings of the National Academy of Sciences **17**(107), 7898–7903 (2010)
42. Loukides, G., Gkoulalas-Divanis, A., Malin, B.: COAT: Constraint-based anonymization of transactions. KAIS **28**(2), 251–282 (2011)
43. Loukides, G., Gkoulalas-Divanis, A., Shao, J.: Anonymizing transaction data to eliminate sensitive inferences. In: DEXA, pp. 400–415 (2010)
44. Loukides, G., Shao, J.: Capturing data usefulness and privacy protection in k-anonymisation. In: SAC, pp. 370–374 (2007)
45. Loukides, G., Shao, J.: Preventing range disclosure in k-anonymised data. Expert Systems with Applications **38**(4), 4559–4574 (2011)
46. Loukides, G., Tziatzios, A., Shao, J.: Towards preference-constrained -anonymisation. In: DASFAA International Workshop on Privacy- Preserving Data Analysis (PPDA), pp. 231–245 (2009)
47. Machanavajjhala, A., Gehrke, J., Kifer, D., Venkitasubramaniam, M.: l-diversity: Privacy beyond k-anonymity. In: ICDE, p. 24 (2006)
48. Malin, B., Loukides, G., Benitez, K., Clayton, E.: Identifiability in biobanks: models, measures, and mitigation strategies. Human Genetics **130**(3), 383–392 (2011)
49. Meyerson, A., Williams, R.: On the complexity of optimal k-anonymity. In: PODS, pp. 223–228 (2004)
50. National Institutes of Health: Policy for sharing of data obtained in NIH supported or conducted genome-wide association studies. NOT-OD-07-088. 2007.
51. Nergiz, M.E., Clifton, C.: Thoughts on k-anonymization. DKE **63**(3), 622–645 (2007)
52. Ohno-Machado, L., Vinterbo, S., Dreiseitl, S.: Effects of data anonymization by cell suppression on descriptive statistics and predictive modeling performance. Journal of American Medical Informatics Association **9**(6), 115119 (2002)
53. Park, H., Shim, K.: Approximate algorithms for k-anonymity. In: SIGMOD, pp. 67–78 (2007)
54. European Parliament, C.: EU Directive on privacy and electronic communications. http://eur-lex.europa.eu/LexUriServ/LexUriServ.do?uri=CELEX:32002L0058:EN:NOT (2002)
55. Phillips, C., Salas, A., Sanchez, J., et al.: Inferring ancestral origin using a single multiplex assay of ancestry-informative marker snps. Forensic Science International: Genetics **1**, 273–280 (2007)
56. Rodgers, J.: Quality assurance and medical ontologies. Methods of Information in Medicine **45**(3), 267–274 (2006)
57. Rothstein, M., Epps, P.: Ethical and legal implications of pharmacogenomics. Nature Review Genetics **2**, 228–231 (2001)
58. Samarati, P.: Protecting respondents identities in microdata release. TKDE **13**(9), 1010–1027 (2001)
59. Sweeney, L.: k-anonymity: a model for protecting privacy. IJUFKS **10**, 557–570 (2002)
60. Terrovitis, M., Mamoulis, N., Kalnis, P.: Privacy-preserving anonymization of set-valued data. PVLDB **1**(1), 115–125 (2008)

61. Terrovitis, M., Mamoulis, N., Kalnis, P.: Local and global recoding methods for anonymizing set-valued data. VLDB J **20**(1), 83–106 (2011)
62. Texas Department of State Health Services: User manual of texas hospital inpatient discharge public use data file. http://www.dshs.state.tx.us/THCIC/ (2008)
63. Truta, T.M., Campan, A., Meyer, P.: Generating microdata with p -sensitive k -anonymity property. In: Secure Data Management, pp. 124–141 (2007)
64. U.S. Department of Health and Human Services Office for Civil Rights: HIPAA administrative simplification regulation text (2006)
65. Wang, R., Li, Y.F., Wang, X., Tang, H., Zhou, X.: Learning your identity and disease from research papers: information leaks in genome wide association study. In: CCS, pp. 534–544 (2009)
66. Wong, R.C., Li, J., Fu, A., K.Wang: alpha-k-anonymity: An enhanced k-anonymity model for privacy-preserving data publishing. In: KDD, pp. 754–759 (2006)
67. Xiao, X., Tao, Y.: Personalized privacy preservation. In: SIGMOD, pp. 229–240 (2006)
68. Xu, J., Wang, W., Pei, J., Wang, X., Shi, B., Fu, A.W.C.: Utility-based anonymization using local recoding. In: KDD, pp. 785–790 (2006)
69. Xu, Y., Wang, K., Fu, A.W.C., Yu, P.S.: Anonymizing transaction databases for publication. In: KDD, pp. 767–775 (2008)
70. Zerhouni, E.A., Nabel, E.: Protecting aggregate genomic data. Science **322**(5898) (2008)
71. Zhou, X., Peng, B., Li, Y.F., Chen, Y., Tang, H., Wang, X.: To release or not to release: evaluating information leaks in aggregate human-genome data. In: ESORICS, pp. 607–627 (2011)

Chapter 3
Re-identification of Clinical Data Through Diagnosis Information

3.1 Motivation

The discovery of genetic and clinical associations is an integral facet of personalized medicine. In this context, researchers need access to large quantities of patient-level data [4], such that various organizations have established data warehouses tied to biorepositories [2]. At the same time, organizations are increasingly required to share patient data beyond their borders. In fact, scientists agree that understanding disease depends on the broad availability of such shared data [11]. For example, in the United States, the National Institutes of Health (NIH) mandates that data collected or analyzed under NIH-sponsored Genome Wide Association Studies (GWAS) is made publicly available in resources, such as the DataBase of Genotype and Phenotype (dbGaP)[8]. Meanwhile, in Europe, there are more than 250 biorepositories, a catalogue of which is accessible through the web.[1]

To address privacy concerns [10] and ensure compliance with regulations, policies that limit the sharing of patient-specific genomic data in a personally identifiable form are emerging. For instance, the NIH recently specified that data submitted to dbGaP should adhere to data sharing regulations, akin to the HIPAA Privacy Rule [17]. The latter rule describes guidelines for privacy protection, such as removing a number of identifying attributes, including patient names and Social Security Numbers, from sensitive biomedical data. In addition, modifying the values of *quasi-identifiers*, which in combination can associate an individual with their published record and sensitive information, using generalization or suppression [14, 16], has also been proposed.

While patient demographics and visits (i.e, whether or not a patient has visited a healthcare provider) are known to act as quasi-identifiers [9, 14], in this chapter, we illustrate that clinical features released in the form of diagnosis codes can also

---

[1] http://www.bbmri.eu/index.php/catalog-of-european-biobanks

A. Gkoulalas-Divanis and G. Loukides, *Anonymization of Electronic Medical Records to Support Clinical Analysis*, SpringerBriefs in Electrical and Computer Engineering, DOI 10.1007/978-1-4614-5668-1_3, © The Author(s) 2013

a

Name	Diagnoses
Jim	493.00
Jack	493.00
Mary	401.0 401.1
Anne	401.1 401.2 401.3
Tom	571.40 571.42
Greg	571.40 571.43

b

Diagnoses	DNA
493.00	CT...A
401.0 401.1	AC...T
571.40 571.42	GC...A

c

Diagnoses	DNA
(401.0,401.1,493.00)	CT...A
(401.0,401.1,493.00)	AC...T
571.40, 571.42	GC...A

Fig. 3.1 An example of: (**a**) original dataset containing patient names and diagnosis codes, (**b**) a de-identified sample of this dataset, and (**c**) a generalized sample of this dataset

facilitate privacy violations. This is due, in part, to the fact that diagnosis codes reside in sources external to the released data, such as the identified electronic medical record (EMR) systems from where they were derived.

Consider, for example, Fig. 3.1a, which illustrates an identified, transaction dataset containing EMR data for a number of patients. Each transaction corresponds to a different patient, and contains all of their ICD codes[2] (we will use the terms ICD and diagnosis codes, interchangeably). A de-identified dataset containing all the diagnosis codes of *Jim*, *Mary*, and *Tom*, as well as their DNA sequences, is shown in Fig. 3.1b. Observe that releasing the latter dataset to support a GWAS may allow an attacker, who has access to the data of Fig. 3.1a, to uniquely associate *Tom* and *Mary* with their DNA sequences. This is possible, because the set of diagnosis codes for these patients appears just once in the identified EMR data of Fig. 3.1a.

It is worth noting that this attack differs from the identity and semantic information disclosure attacks that were discussed in Sects. 2.1 and 2.2, respectively. In the attack we consider, the published dataset does not necessarily contain the records of all patients, whose information is contained in the EMR system, and that each published record contains a DNA sequence that is not contained in the identified EMR dataset. This is because, it is often the case that the data of a selected subset of patients are useful in the context of GWAS and that the patients' DNA sequences are not accessible to all users of the EMR system [12]. In addition, we assume that an attacker does not know whether or not a patient's record is contained in the published dataset. This assumption models the so-called *journalist scenario* [3], in which membership of the record in the sample is difficult to determine (e.g., when a small percentage of EMRs in a population are released). We will study different scenarios, in which this assumption is waived, in Chap. 4.

We emphasize that this attack is realistic, since diagnosis codes are increasingly disseminated in sources including bio-repositories and publicly available hospital discharge datasets [14], and poses a serious privacy threat. This is because, when this attack succeeds, patients become associated with all their diagnosis codes and genetic information, which may be misused or abused [13]. However, existing

---

[2]We refer to ICD-9 codes, which are used to assign health insurance billing codes to diagnoses in the United States.

privacy regulations and research methodologies are not designed to deal with diagnosis codes residing in EMR systems, and focus on data with simpler semantics, such as identifying and demographic information.

To model this attack, we will first describe the type of the datasets we consider in Sect. 3.2. Then, we present a measure to quantify the risk of re-identification, based on diagnosis codes, and demonstrate its application on an Electronic Medical Record (EMR) dataset from Vanderbilt University Medical Center, in Sect. 3.3. Last, in Sect. 3.4, we turn our attention to measures that capture the loss of utility entailed by anonymization when sharing patients records.

3.2 Structure of the Datasets Used in the Attack

Following the notation that was presented in Chap. 2, we consider a dataset $\mathscr{D}_P$ that contains $|\mathscr{D}_P|$ transactions. Each transaction T in $\mathscr{D}_P$ corresponds to a different patient and is represented as a tuple $\langle ID, I \rangle$, where ID is a unique identifier for T (e.g., a patient's name), and I is an itemset. I is comprised of diagnosis codes, which are derived from the domain $\mathscr{I}$ of ICD codes. For example, the dataset shown in Fig. 3.1a contains six transactions, the first of which has $ID = Jim$ and $I = \{493.00\}$. Also, $\mathscr{D}_S$ is a dataset that contains $|\mathscr{D}_S|$ records of the form $\langle I, DNA \rangle$. I is an itemset comprised of the diagnosis codes of a patient and DNA is this patient's DNA sequence. We assume that there is an one-to-one mapping between every transaction in $\mathscr{D}_S$ and a transaction in $\mathscr{D}_P$. That is, $\mathscr{D}_P$ models the entire set of patient records (population), and $\mathscr{D}_S$ the de-identified sample, which contains patient diagnosis codes and DNA sequences and is to be shared to support GWAS.

3.3 Distinguishability Measure and Its Application to EMR Data

A measure, called *distinguishability* (*dis*), was proposed by Loukides et al. [6] to capture the risk of associating patients in the dataset $\mathscr{D}_S$, based on their diagnosis information that is contained in $\mathscr{D}_P$. The following definition illustrates the distinguishability measure.

Definition 3.1 (Distinguishability (dis)). Given a record $T = \langle I, DNA \rangle$ in $\mathscr{D}_S$, we define the *distinguishability* (*dis*) of T as the number of records in $\mathscr{D}_P$ that have exactly the same I with T.

Distinguishability takes values in $[1, |\mathscr{D}_P|]$ and, given a record $T = \langle I, DNA \rangle$ in $\mathscr{D}_S$, it holds that $dis(T) = sup(I, \mathscr{D}_P)$. Using this notation, a patient represented with T in $\mathscr{D}_S$ is *uniquely identifiable* when $dis(T) = 1$, while larger distinguishability values imply higher privacy. For example, the distinguishability of the first record in

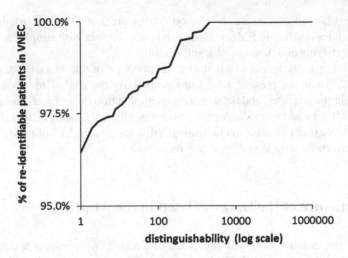

Fig. 3.2 Percentage of patient records in *VNEC* that are vulnerable to re-identification when data are released in their original form [6]

the dataset of Fig. 3.1b is 2, because the diagnosis code 493.00 is supported by the first two records in the dataset of Fig. 3.1a. On the other hand, the distinguishability for the second record in the dataset of Fig. 3.1b is 1, hence *Mary* is uniquely identifiable. Note that distinguishability equals the inverse of the probability of associating an individual to their record in $\mathscr{D}_S$, based on *all* the diagnosis codes of a record in $\mathscr{D}_S$.

Based on distinguishability, the level of protection offered by a dataset $\mathscr{D}_S$ from an attacker, who uses a dataset $\mathscr{D}_P$, can be measured based on the distribution of *dis* values, for all records in $\mathscr{D}_S$. Figure 3.2, for example, which was borrowed from [6], illustrates the distinguishability scores for an EMR dataset. *VNEC* stands for *Vanderbilt Native Electrical Conduction* and contains 2,762 records, one for each patient. This dataset is related to a GWAS on native electrical conduction within the ventricles of the heart and is derived from the de-identified version of the EMR system of the Vanderbilt University Medical Center [15]. The latter is referred to as *Vanderbilt Population* (*VP*) dataset and contains 1.17*M* records. As can be seen in Fig. 3.2, over 96 % of records in *VNEC* had *dis* = 1, and thus were uniquely re-identifiable. For more details on the construction of *VNEC* and *VP* datasets, and further discussion of the adversarial knowledge that is assumed and the application scenario, we refer the reader to [6].

To explain the high distinguishability scores of Fig. 3.2, it worths considering the characteristics of *VNEC*, which are summarized in Table 3.1 together with Fig. 3.3 below. As can be seen, the majority of diagnosis codes in *VNEC* appear a small number of times (e.g., 38 % of codes appear at most ten times), while a patient's record contains only 3.1 out of 5.8*K* possible diagnosis codes, on average. Thus, it is unlikely for two records in *VNEC* to have the same set of diagnosis codes. At the same time, a patient in *VP* is associated with only 3 out of 13.5*K* records.

Table 3.1 Description of the *VNEC* dataset

Dataset	N	$|\mathscr{I}|$	Max. number of ICD codes per record	Avg. number of ICD codes per record
VNEC	2,762	5,830	25	3.1
VP	1,174,793	13,538	370	3

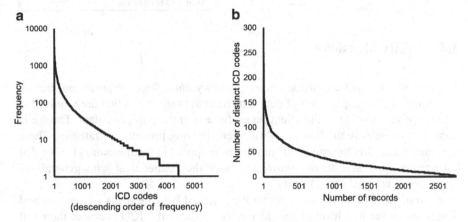

Fig. 3.3 Characteristics of the *VNEC* dataset: (**a**) frequency of the ICD codes, and (**b**) number of ICD codes per record

This implies that a record in *VNEC* shares the same set of diagnosis codes with only a very small number on records in the *VP* dataset, although this dataset is much larger than *VNEC*.

It is important to note that the distribution of *dis* values is affected by applying suppression and generalization. Computing the *distinguishability* of the records in a suppressed dataset $\mathscr{D}_S$ is straightforward, as we simply disregard all diagnosis codes that have been suppressed. Assuming, for instance, that we have suppressed the diagnosis code 401.0 from the dataset of Fig. 3.1b, the distinguishability of the second record in this dataset increases to 2. In the case of generalization, distinguishability can be measured after transforming the diagnosis codes in $\mathscr{D}_P$, based on the way they were transformed in $\mathscr{D}_S$. Note that the dataset that results from transforming $\mathscr{D}_P$ is used only for the calculation of distinguishability, and it is not published. As an example, consider the dataset shown in Fig. 3.1c, in which the diagnosis codes 401.0, 401.1, and 493.00 have been replaced with (401.0, 401.1, 493.00), which is interpreted as any non-empty subset of these codes. To compute the distinguishability of the first record in the latter dataset, we need to transform the dataset shown in Fig. 3.1a by replacing all the instances of these diagnosis codes with (401.0, 401.1., 493.00), as shown in Fig. 3.4. Since (401.0, 401.1, 493.00) is contained in four records of the dataset of Fig. 3.4, the distinguishability of the first record in the dataset of Fig. 3.1b is 4.

Fig. 3.4 The result of
replacing 401.0, 401.1, and
493.00, in the dataset of
Fig. 3.1a, with
(401.0,401.1,493.00)

Name	Diagnoses
Jim	(401.0,401.1,493.00)
Jack	(401.0,401.1,493.00)
Mary	(401.0,401.1,493.00)
Anne	(401.0,401.1,493.00)401.2401.3
Tom	571.40571.42
Greg	571.40571.43

3.4 Utility Measures

The protection of patient privacy is a regulatory and ethical requirement, but, at the same time, the application of data transformation strategies that are required to achieve privacy may limit the scientific usefulness of the published data. Thus, it is important to measure the loss in utility when applying protection strategies. There are many data utility measures that have been proposed in the literature [1, 5, 14, 16] but are not applicable to our setting, because they either deal with generalized [1, 14, 16] or nominal data [1] only.

To examine data utility, we consider the standard ICD hierarchy of diseases and diagnoses. In the leaf level of this hierarchy, we have the ICD codes in their full (five-digit) form. A number of these codes have three-digit disease codes (called *categories*) as their ascendants, and categories are organized into 120 *sections*, which lie in the third level of the hierarchy. Sections are further organized into 17 *chapters*, which lie in the fourth level of the hierarchy. The root of this hierarchy is the most general term *any diagnosis code*. As an example, consider Fig. 3.5, which illustrates the five-digit code 250.02 and its ascendants according to the ICD hierarchy. This code denotes "diabetes mellitus, type II, uncontrolled, without complication", and its ascendants in ascending order are: the category 250, which denotes "diabetes mellitus, type II", the section "diseases of other endocrine glands", the chapter "endocrine, nutritional, metabolic, immunity", and the root of the hierarchy "any diagnosis code".

Data utility can be measured either as an aggregated score of the anonymized dataset, or at a record-level. To evaluate the utility of an anonymized dataset containing diagnosis codes, one can resort to measuring the percent of retained diagnoses at different levels of the hierarchy [6]. Intuitively, retaining a small percentage of diagnosis codes, after applying suppression, may indicate a significant loss of utility.

Although the use of this statistic can be a good starting point for evaluating data utility, certain tasks are difficult or even impossible to perform when the majority of diagnosis codes at a five-digit or three-digit level are suppressed to preserve privacy. For instance, consider a dataset in which all five-level ICD codes, whose ascendant is the three-digit level code 250 denoting "diabetes mellitus type II". This dataset is not useful for measuring the number of patients having "diabetes mellitus type II",

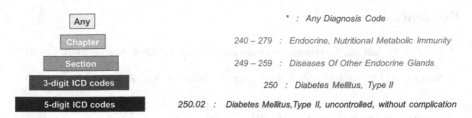

Fig. 3.5 The five-digit code 250.02 and its ascendants at different levels of the ICD hierarchy

but it still allows counting the number of patients diagnosed with "diseases of other endocrine glands", when all other diagnosis codes belonging in this section of the ICD hierarchy are published. Thus, the descriptions of the retained diagnosis codes at the various levels of aggregation indicate whether the data remain useful or not.

The *Size Loss* (*SL*) and *Relative Size Loss* (*RSL*) measures quantify the loss of data utility that is incurred by suppression, at a record level. The following definitions explain the *SL* and *RSL* measures.

Definition 3.2 (Size Loss (SL)). Given a dataset $\mathscr{D}_S = \{T_1, \ldots, T_N\}$ and a version $\tilde{\mathscr{D}}_S = \{\tilde{T}_1, \ldots, \tilde{T}_N\}$ of it, from which some diagnosis codes have been suppressed, the *Size Loss* equals $\sum_{\forall T \in \mathscr{D}_S} |I| - \sum_{\forall \tilde{T} \in \tilde{\mathscr{D}}_S} |\tilde{I}|$, where $|I|$ and $|\tilde{I}|$ denotes the number of diagnosis codes contained in a record in $\mathscr{D}_S$ and $\tilde{\mathscr{D}}_S$, respectively.

Definition 3.3 (Relative Size Loss (RSL)). Given a dataset $\mathscr{D}_S = \{T_1, \ldots, T_N\}$ and a version $\tilde{\mathscr{D}}_S = \{\tilde{T}_1, \ldots, \tilde{T}_N\}$ of it, from which some diagnosis codes have been suppressed, the *Relative Size Loss* equals $1 - \frac{\sum_{\forall \tilde{T} \in \tilde{\mathscr{D}}_S} |\tilde{I}|}{\sum_{\forall T \in \mathscr{D}_S} |I|}$, where $|I|$ and $|\tilde{I}|$ denotes the number of diagnosis codes contained in a record in $\mathscr{D}_S$ and $\tilde{\mathscr{D}}_S$, respectively.

Both *SL* and *RSL* measure how suppression affects the distribution of diagnosis codes, although in different ways. Specifically, *SL* captures the difference between the size of sets I and $\tilde{I}$, for all records in $\mathscr{D}_S$, before and after applying suppression to it, while *RSL* measures the fraction of diagnosis codes that are removed from $\mathscr{D}_S$ during suppression. As an example of computing the *SL* and *RSL* measures, consider suppressing the diagnosis code 401.1 from the second record of the dataset shown in Fig. 3.1b. In this case, the *SL* and *RSL* measures are computed as $2 - 1 = 1$ and $1 - \frac{1}{2} = 0.5$, respectively.

Finally, it can be the case that data publishers regard only certain diagnosis codes as useful for an intended analytic task, but choose to publish additional codes in order to help studies that are unknown to them and to generally promote data re-use efforts [7]. In this case, the aforementioned utility measures should be applied only to the diagnosis codes that are deemed as useful.

References

1. Agrawal, R., Srikant, R.: Privacy-preserving data mining. SIGMOD Record **29**(2), 439–450 (2000)
2. Barbour, V.: Uk biobank: A project in search of a protocol? Lancet **361**(9370), 1734–1738 (2003)
3. Emam, K.E.: Methods for the de-identification of electronic health records for genomic research. Genome Medicine **3**(4), 25 (2011)
4. Gurwitz, D., Lunshof, J., Altman, R.: A call for the creation of personalized medicine databases. Nature Reviews Drug Discovery **5**(1), 23–26 (2006)
5. Lin, Z., Hewett, M., Altman, R.: Using binning to maintain confidentiality of medical data. In: AMIA Annual Symposium, pp. 454–458 (2002)
6. Loukides, G., Denny, J., Malin, B.: The disclosure of diagnosis codes can breach research participants' privacy. Journal of the American Medical Informatics Association **17**, 322–327 (2010)
7. Loukides, G., Gkoulalas-Divanis, A., Malin, B.: Anonymization of electronic medical records for validating genome-wide association studies. Proceedings of the National Academy of Sciences **17**(107), 7898–7903 (2010)
8. Mailman, M., Feolo, M., Jin, Y., Kimura, M., Tryka, K., Bagoutdinov, R., et al.: The ncbi dbgap database of genotypes and phenotypes. Nature Genetics **39**, 1181–1186 (2007)
9. Malin, B.: A computational model to protect patient data from location-based re-identification. Artificial Intelligence in Medicine **40**, 223–239 (2007)
10. McGuire, A., Fisher, R., Cusenza, P., et al.: Confidentiality, privacy, and security of genetic and genomic text information in electronic health records: points to consider. Genetics in Medicine **10**(7), 495–499 (2008)
11. Organization for Economic Co-operation and Development, Directorate for Science, Technology and Industry: Towards a global biological resource centre network. http://www.oecd.org/document/51/0,3746,en_2649_34537_33791027_1_1_1_1,00.html (2007)
12. Roden, D., Pulley, J., Basford, M., Bernard, G., Clayton, E., Balser, J., Masys, D.: Development of a large scale de-identified dna biobank to enable personalized medicine. Clinical Pharmacology and Therapeutics **84**(3), 362–369 (2008)
13. Rothstein, M., Epps, P.: Ethical and legal implications of pharmacogenomics. Nature Review Genetics **2**, 228–231 (2001)
14. Samarati, P.: Protecting respondents identities in microdata release. TKDE **13**(9), 1010–1027 (2001)
15. Stead, W., Bates, R., Byrd, J., Giuse, D., Miller, R., Shultz, E.: Case study: The vanderbilt university medical center information management architecture (2003)
16. Sweeney, L.: k-anonymity: a model for protecting privacy. IJUFKS **10**, 557–570 (2002)
17. U.S. Department of Health and Human Services, Office for Civil Rights: Standards for protection of electronic health information; final rule (2003). Federal Register, 45 CFR: Pt. 164

Chapter 4
Preventing Re-identification While Supporting GWAS

4.1 Motivation

Electronic medical record (EMR) systems are increasingly recognized as an important resource for GWAS [12]. They contain detailed patient-level data on large populations, incorporate demographics and standardized clinical terminologies, and can reduce both costs and time of conducting large-scale GWAS. To support GWAS, EMR data are often combined with genomic data and disseminated in a de-identified form. However, as explained in Chap. 3, publishing these data may lead to re-identification, because it is possible for an attacker to link patient identities with their published EMR data, using the diagnosis codes contained in external, identified data sources (e.g., hospital discharge databases or the original EMR system).

Since publishing the diagnosis codes is essential to supporting GWAS, the diagnosis codes should be disseminated in a manner that mitigates the aforementioned re-identification threat. This can be achieved by (i) specifying the sets of diagnosis codes that are potentially linkable to identified data sources, and (ii) modifying the linkable diagnosis codes so that the patient records containing these codes can be linked to a sufficiently large number of individuals, based on these codes. Diagnosis code modification can prevent the linkage of a patient to their DNA sequence, but, at the same time, it may distort the associations between sets of codes corresponding to GWAS-related diseases and the DNA sequence. Therefore, it is crucial to retain the ability to support clinical association validations when modifying clinical profiles.

Anonymizing diagnosis codes is a challenging computational problem, because a small number among thousands of possible diagnosis codes are assigned to a patient. Thus, these data are difficult to anonymize without excessive information loss [1]. This implies that anonymization algorithms that have been designed for demographics [3, 7, 15–17], such as those described in Chap. 2, are not adequate to deal with the problem of publishing diagnosis codes. Algorithms for anonymizing transaction data can be applied to high-dimensional and sparse datasets, as discussed

A. Gkoulalas-Divanis and G. Loukides, *Anonymization of Electronic Medical Records to Support Clinical Analysis*, SpringerBriefs in Electrical and Computer Engineering, DOI 10.1007/978-1-4614-5668-1_4, © The Author(s) 2013

in Chap. 2. However, these algorithms have the following shortcomings that may significantly affect the level of both privacy and utility of the published data.

- First, they are limited in the specification of privacy requirements. For instance, potentially linkable combinations of diagnosis codes may involve certain codes only and may vary in size, but existing approaches attempt to protect all combinations of a certain number of codes [18, 19]. In this case, these approaches would unnecessarily incur excessive information loss [9, 10]. Worse, employing ρ-uncertainty [2] may not prevent re-identification, which is a legal requirement for publishing GWAS-related data [13].
- Second, they do not allow data publishers to specify data utility requirements, such as that the published data needs to guarantee the validation of specific GWAS. Thus, they may produce data that is useless for the purpose of supporting GWAS.
- Third, they adopt data transformation strategies that are ineffective at minimizing information loss. For example, the approach of Xu et al. [20] uses a global suppression model, which may result in significant loss of data utility, while the works of Terrovitis et al. [18, 19] and He et al. [6] adopt the hierarchy-based generalization model that does not allow exploring a large part of possible generalizations.

In this chapter, we discuss an approach that prevents data linkage attacks via diagnosis codes, while ensuring that the released data remain useful for GWAS validation [5, 9]. In summary, this approach extracts a privacy policy in the form of sets of diagnosis codes that require protection and anonymizes each record that contains any of these codes to ensure it links to no less than k individuals with respect to these sets. Anonymization is achieved by replacing diagnosis codes with sets of semantically related codes to satisfy a utility policy, which reflects the distribution of GWAS-related diseases to be preserved. For instance, when applied to the dataset shown in Fig. 4.1a, with $k = 5$ and the utility policy of Fig. 4.1c, the approach of [5, 9] extracts the privacy policy of Fig. 4.1d, and generates the dataset of Fig. 4.1e. The latter satisfies the privacy requirements because each record links to no less than five individuals with respect to the sets of ICD codes in the privacy policy, as well as utility because the associations between diseases and DNA sequences are unaffected; i.e., the distribution of the GWAS-related diseases is preserved. For example, there are 6, 5, and 8 patients suffering *asthma, prostate cancer*, and *pancreatic cancer* in either of the datasets shown in Fig. 4.1a, e, respectively.

4.2 Background

In what follows, we define the structure of the considered datasets, as well as the notions of privacy and utility policies. We also present a strategy to anonymize diagnosis codes and a measure to capture information loss incurred by anonymization.

a

ID	Diagnoses	DNA
1	493.00 493.01 493.02	CT...A
2	157.0 157.1 157.2 157.3 185	GC...A
3	157.0 157.1 157.9	CA...A
4	157.1 157.2 493.00 493.02	CG...T
5	157.0 157.1 157.2 185	AC...A
6	157.0 185 493.00 493.01	CC...A
7	157.1 493.00 493.02	TA...T
8	157.0 185 493.00 493.02	GC...C
9	157.0 157.3 185 493.01	AA...G

b

ID	Name	Service Date	Diagnoses
1	Jim	01/02/08	493.00 493.01 493.02
2	Mary	01/02/08	157.0 185
2	Mary	07/09/09	157.1 157.2 157.3
3	Bob	03/08/08	157.9
3	Bob	07/09/09	157.0 157.1
4	Anne	07/09/09	157.1 157.2 493.00 493.02
5	Alice	03/08/08	157.0 185
5	Alice	07/09/09	157.1 157.2
6	Tom	01/02/08	493.00 493.01
6	Tom	03/08/08	157.0 185
7	Steve	01/02/08	493.00
7	Steve	03/08/08	493.02
7	Steve	07/09/09	157.1
8	David	01/02/08	493.00 157.0
8	David	03/08/08	493.02 185
9	Ellen	01/02/08	157.0 185
9	Ellen	03/08/08	493.01
9	Ellen	07/09/09	157.3

c

Diagnoses	Disease
493.00 493.01 493.02	Asthma
185	Prostate cancer
157.0 157.1 157.2 157.3 157.9	Pancreatic cancer

d

Diagnoses	Support
157.1 157.2 157.3	1
157.9	1
493.00 493.01 493.02	1

e

ID	Diagnoses	DNA
1	(493.00, 493.01, 493.02)	CT...A
2	(157.0, 157.1, 157.2, 157.3, 157.9) (185)	GC...A
3	(157.0, 157.1, 157.2, 157.3, 157.9)	CA...A
4	(157.0, 157.1, 157.2, 157.3, 157.9) (493.00, 493.01, 493.02)	CG...T
5	(157.0, 157.1, 157.2, 157.3, 157.9) (185)	AC...A
6	(157.0, 157.1, 157.2, 157.3, 157.9) (185) (493.00, 493.01, 493.02)	CC...A
7	(157.0, 157.1, 157.2, 157.3, 157.9) (493.00, 493.01, 493.02)	TA...T
8	(157.0, 157.1, 157.2, 157.3, 157.9) (185) (493.00, 493.01, 493.02)	GC...C
9	(157.0, 157.1, 157.2, 157.3, 157.9) (185) (493.00, 493.01, 493.02)	AA...G

Fig. 4.1 Biomedical datasets (fictional) and policies employed by the proposed anonymization approach: (**a**) research data, (**b**) identified EMR data, (**c**) utility policy (**d**) privacy policy, and (**e**) a five-anonymization for the research data

4.2.1 Structure of the Data

We consider two types of datasets. The first dataset is denoted with $\mathscr{D}$ and corresponds to the GWAS-related dataset that is to be published. Each transaction in $\mathscr{D}$ corresponds to a different patient and is a tuple $\langle I, DNA \rangle$, where I is the patient's set of ICD codes and DNA their genomic sequence. The second dataset $\mathscr{E}$

contains data derived from an identified EMR system. It contains patients' *explicit identifiers* (e.g., personal names), service dates, and a set of ICD codes. Each record in $\mathcal{E}$ is a triple $\langle ID, ServDate, I \rangle$ and it represents the set of diagnosis codes that were assigned to a patient during a visit on a specific date. Note that a patient may be associated with multiple records in $\mathcal{E}$, each having a different *ServDate*. Examples of $\mathcal{D}$ and $\mathcal{E}$ are depicted in Fig. 4.1a, b, respectively. To protect privacy, an anonymized version $\tilde{\mathcal{D}}$ of $\mathcal{D}$ can be constructed. Each record of $\tilde{\mathcal{D}}$ contains a patient's anonymized diagnosis codes and their DNA sequence.

4.2.2 Privacy and Utility Policies

To capture data publishers' privacy requirements, the authors of [5, 9] proposed the notion of privacy policy and its satisfiability. These notions are illustrated below.

Definition 4.1 (Privacy policy). Given a dataset $\mathcal{D}$, a *privacy policy* $\mathcal{P}$ is defined as a set of *privacy constraints*. Each privacy constraint $p \in \mathcal{P}$ is a non-empty set of diagnosis codes in $\mathcal{I}$, which is *supported* when $sup(p, \mathcal{D}) > 0$, and *non-supported* otherwise.

Definition 4.2 (Privacy policy satisfiability). Given a parameter k, a privacy constraint $p = \{i_1, \ldots, i_r\} \in \mathcal{P}$ is *satisfied* when the itemset in $\tilde{\mathcal{D}}$ that is comprised of all items in p is: (1) supported by at least k transactions in $\tilde{\mathcal{D}}$, or (2) non-supported in $\tilde{\mathcal{D}}$ and each of its proper subsets is either supported by at least k transactions in $\tilde{\mathcal{D}}$ or is non-supported in $\tilde{\mathcal{D}}$. $\mathcal{P}$ is satisfied when every $p \in \mathcal{P}$ is satisfied.

As an example, consider the privacy policy of Fig. 4.1d, the dataset of Fig. 4.1e and $k = 5$. It can be seen that the privacy constraint $\{157.9\}$ is *supported* in the dataset of Fig. 4.1e. This privacy constraint is also *satisfied* for $k = 5$ in the same dataset because all of its non-empty subsets, which in this case is only the privacy constraint itself, appear in at least five records. Due to the fact that all privacy constraints of Fig. 4.1d are satisfied in the dataset of Fig. 4.1e, the privacy policy is satisfied.

The satisfaction of the privacy policy prevents patient re-identification because an attacker cannot use potentially linkable sets of ICD codes to link a DNA sequence to less than k patients in the released dataset $\tilde{\mathcal{D}}$. In other words, the probability of re-identification remains always at least $1/k$.

Privacy protection is offered at the expense of data utility [7, 17], and thus it is important to ensure that anonymized data remain useful for the intended task. The approaches discussed in Chap. 2 attempt to achieve this by minimizing the amount of information loss incurred when anonymizing transaction data [6, 18, 20], but do not guarantee furnishing a useful result for intended applications. By contrast, the methodology presented in this chapter offers such guarantees through the introduction of utility policies.

Definition 4.3 (Utility policy and its satisfiability). A utility policy $\mathcal{U}$ is defined as a set of *diseases*, each referred to as a *utility constraint*. A utility constraint $u \in \mathcal{U}$ is *satisfied* when $sup(u, \tilde{\mathcal{D}})$ equals the number of transactions in $\mathcal{D}$ that support at least one of the ICD codes contained in u. A utility policy is *satisfied* if all of its utility constraints are satisfied.

Thus, the number of transactions in $\mathcal{D}$ that support any item contained in a utility constraint $u \in \mathcal{U}$ can be accurately computed from the anonymized dataset $\tilde{\mathcal{D}}$, when u is satisfied and all items in u have been generalized. This is crucial in supporting GWAS, where the support of *diseases* (i.e., number of patients associated with any of the diagnosis codes referring to a disease) needs to be determined. Similarly, satisfying a utility policy ensures that the distribution of diseases contained in this policy will not be affected by anonymization. This allows all associations between diseases and DNA sequences present in the original dataset to be preserved in the anonymized dataset.

Consider, for example, the utility policy of Fig. 4.1c, and the utility constraint *asthma* corresponding to the set of ICD codes $\{493.00, 493.01, 493.02\}$. The latter constraint is satisfied, since the number of patients suffering from *asthma* in the dataset of Fig. 4.1e (i.e., the records harboring $(493.00, 493.01, 493.02)$) is equal to the number of patients harboring at least one of the ICD codes related to *asthma* in the dataset of Fig. 4.1a. Similarly, it can be verified that the utility constraints for *prostate cancer* and *pancreatic cancer* are satisfied as well; therefore, the utility policy of Fig. 4.1c is satisfied.

4.2.3 Anonymization Strategy

Loukides et al. [9] proposed an anonymization strategy that creates an anonymized dataset $\tilde{D}$ from $\mathcal{D}$ by replacing every ICD code in $\mathcal{I}$ with a unique *anonymized item*. An anonymized item is represented as a set of ICD codes and interpreted as any non-empty subset of the codes it contains. Disparate anonymized codes are mutually exclusive, such that there are no ICD codes in multiple anonymized items. The process of replacing ICD codes with anonymized items is explained in the following definition [9].

Definition 4.4 (Anonymization Strategy). The anonymized dataset $\tilde{\mathcal{D}}$ is derived from $\mathcal{D}$ in two steps by:

1. Constructing a new set $\tilde{\mathcal{I}}$ such that: (i) each ICD code in $\mathcal{I}$ is uniquely mapped to an *anonymized item* $\tilde{i} \in \tilde{\mathcal{I}}$ that is a subset of $\mathcal{I}$, and (ii) $\mathcal{I} = \left(\bigcup_{m=1}^{|\tilde{\mathcal{I}}|} \tilde{i_m} \right) \cup \mathbf{S}$, where $|\tilde{\mathcal{I}}|$ denotes the size of $\tilde{\mathcal{I}}$ and $\mathbf{S}$ the set of suppressed ICD codes from $\mathcal{I}$, and
2. Replacing each ICD code i in $\mathcal{D}$ with the anonymized item this code has been mapped to, if i has been mapped to a non-empty subset of $\mathcal{I}$, or suppressing i otherwise.

Consider, for example, applying the anonymization strategy to the dataset of Fig. 4.1a to derive the anonymized dataset of Fig. 4.1e. To create $\tilde{I}$, ICD codes 493.00, 493.01 and 493.02 are mapped to an anonymized item $\tilde{i}_1 = (493.00, 493.01, 493.02)$, the ICD codes 157.0, 157.1, 157.2, 157.3 and 157.9 are mapped to $\tilde{i}_2 = (157.0, 157.1, 157.2, 157.3, 157.9)$ and the ICD code 185 is mapped to $\tilde{i}_3 = (185)$. Since no ICD code is suppressed, we have $\tilde{I} = \tilde{i}_1 \cup \tilde{i}_2 \cup \tilde{i}_3$. Subsequently, the dataset shown in Fig. 4.1e is derived by replacing each of the ICD codes in D with the anonymized item $\tilde{i}_1$, $\tilde{i}_2$ or $\tilde{i}_3$ this ICD code has been mapped to.

The aforementioned anonymization strategy may replace ICD codes with semantically consistent, but more general terms, typically specified by hierarchies [16, 17] or, by default, the ICD coding hierarchy.[1] Alternatively, ICD codes may also be suppressed. As we explain later, this occurs when generalization does not suffice to satisfy the specified privacy policy. Both generalization and suppression effectively increase the number of patients to which a privacy constraint is associated, thereby reducing the risk of re-identification.

Notably, the way diagnosis codes are generalized eliminates the need of hierarchies and allows the production of more fine-grained anonymizations with substantially better utility than those constructed by alternative generalization strategies [18, 20]. As an example, consider *diabetes mellitus type-2*, a disease that is associated with a set of ICD codes of the form 250.xy, where x is an integer in $[0, 9]$ and $y \in \{0, 2\}$. The existing algorithms that employ hierarchy-based generalization models [4, 18, 19] would replace any set of this type of code with 250 (denoting *diabetes mellitus*) when a hierarchy that associates five-digit ICD codes to their three-digit counterparts is applied. By doing so, the generalization process makes it impossible to distinguish between *diabetes mellitus type-1* and *type-2*, and yield anonymized data that is meaningless for validating GWAS on *diabetes mellitus type-2*. In contrast, the anonymization strategy of [9] allows a utility constraint corresponding to *diabetes mellitus type-2* to be specified and guarantees that the number of patients diagnosed with *diabetes mellitus type-2* will be equal in the original and anonymized clinical profiles, when this utility constraint is satisfied. This effectively preserves all associations between this disease and DNA regions and, thus, allows for validation of GWAS studies, as explained in [9].

4.2.4 Information Loss Measure

Both generalization and suppression incur information loss that needs to be controlled to help the utility of anonymized data. Observe that the amount of information loss depends on (i) the number of transactions in $\mathcal{D}$ that support the ICD code that is to be generalized (i.e., generalizing a frequent ICD code incurs a large amount of information loss), (ii) the number of ICD codes that are generalized together (i.e., mapping a large number of ICD codes to the same anonymized

---

[1] http://www.cdc.gov/nchs/icd/icd9cm.htm

item incurs a large amount of information loss because the anonymized item is difficult to be interpreted), and (iii) the semantic distance of the ICD codes that are generalized together (i.e., generalizing ICD codes together that are not semantically related incurs high information loss). Thus, the authors of [5] propose the following measure that takes all these factors into consideration.

Definition 4.5 (Information Loss). The *Information Loss* (*IL*) for an anonymized item $\tilde{i}_m$ is defined as

$$IL(\tilde{i}_m) = \frac{2^{|\tilde{i}_m|} - 1}{2^M - 1} \times w(\tilde{i}_m) \times \frac{sup(\tilde{i}_m, \tilde{\mathscr{D}})}{N}$$

where $|\tilde{i}_m|$ denotes the number of ICD codes that are mapped to $\tilde{i}_m$, M is the number of ICD codes in $\mathscr{I}$, N is the number of transactions in $\mathscr{D}$, and $w : \tilde{\mathscr{I}} \rightarrow [0, 1]$ is a function assigning a weight to $\tilde{i}_m$ based on the semantical distance of the ICD codes it contains. We compute this distance following [14] and using the ICD coding hierarchy.

To illustrate how the above measure can be computed, consider the ICD codes 493.00, 493.01 and 493.02 in the dataset of Fig. 4.1a, which are mapped to the anonymized item $\tilde{i}_1 = (493.00, 493.01, 493.02)$ in the data of Fig. 4.1e, and a weight of 0.375. Using *IL*, the information loss of this generalization can be computed as $IL(\tilde{i}_1) = \frac{2^3 - 1}{2^9 - 1} \times 0.375 \times \frac{6}{9} \approx 0.0034$. Similarly, using the same weight, the information loss incurred by mapping 157.0, 157.1, 157.2, 157.3 and 157.9 to $\tilde{i}_2 = (157.0, 157.1, 157.2, 157.3, 157.9)$ can be calculated as $IL(\tilde{i}_2) = 0.0072$. Notice that the latter generalization incurs a higher amount of information loss, since $\tilde{i}_2$ is comprised of a larger number of ICD codes than that of $\tilde{i}_1$ and is associated with a larger number of patients in the anonymized dataset.

4.3 Algorithms for Anonymizing Diagnosis Codes

In this section, we begin by discussing an algorithm for extracting privacy policies that was proposed in [9]. Then, we provide an overview of two algorithms for anonymizing diagnosis codes that were proposed in [9] and [5], respectively. The goal of both of these algorithms is to produce anonymizations that guarantee both privacy and help the validation of GWAS.

4.3.1 Privacy Policy Extraction

To allow data owners formulating a privacy policy, the *Privacy Policy Extraction* (PPE) algorithm was proposed by Loukides et al. [9]. This algorithm assumes a scenario in which an attacker knows: (i) a patient's explicit identifiers, (ii) a certain set of ICD codes for each patient, and (iii) whether a patient's record is contained

---

Algorithm 5   PPE($\mathcal{D}, \mathcal{F}, k$) [9]

---

    input: Dataset $\mathcal{D}$, filtering condition $\mathcal{F}$, parameter k
    output: Privacy policy $\mathcal{P}'$
1. $\mathcal{P}' \leftarrow Filter(\mathcal{D}, \mathcal{F}, k)$
2.   Sort the elements of $\mathcal{P}'$ in descending order based on their size
3.   **for each** element p_i in $\mathcal{P}'$, $i = 1, \ldots, N$
4.   **for each** element p_j in $\mathcal{P}'$, $j = i+1, \ldots, N$
5.   **if** all ICDs code in p_j are contained in p_i
6. $\mathcal{P}' \leftarrow \mathcal{P}' \setminus p_j$
7.   **if** $sup(p_i, \mathcal{D}) \geq k$
8. $\mathcal{P}' \leftarrow \mathcal{P} \setminus T_i$
13. **return** $\mathcal{P}'$

---

in $\mathcal{D}$. Knowledge of the first two types can come in the form of background knowledge [11] or may be solicited by exploiting external data sources, such as publicly available voter lists combined with hospital discharge summaries [16] or the identified electronic medical record (EMR) system available to the primary care environment [8]. Knowledge of the third type can be inferred by applying the procedure used to create the research sample from a larger patient population (e.g., all medical records in an EMR system), which is often described in the literature. Thus, this scenario differs from the one considered in Chap. 3, in which attackers were assumed not to possess knowledge of the third type.

Before presenting the PPE algorithm, we illustrate the notion of *filtering condition*, which was used by Loukides et al. [9] to model potentially identifying ICD codes. Given a parameter k, the application of a filtering condition $\mathcal{F}$ to $\mathcal{D}$, constructs a set of combinations of ICD codes. Specifically, the authors of [9] considered two concrete filtering conditions, namely *single visit* and *all visits*. In the single visit case, it is assumed that the set of ICD codes for each patient's visit is potentially identifying, whereas in the all visits case, all ICD codes of a patient are regarded as potentially identifying. It should also be noted that PPE allows data publishers to use different filtering conditions according to their expectations about which ICD codes are potentially identifying.

Algorithm 5 illustrates the Privacy Policy Extraction (PPE) algorithm. PPE takes as input the original dataset $\mathcal{D}$, a filtering condition $\mathcal{F}$, and a parameter k, and returns a privacy policy. The algorithm begins by applying $\mathcal{F}$ on $\mathcal{D}$, using a function *Filter*. This way a privacy policy $\mathcal{P}'$, which may contain more privacy constraints than necessary to satisfy data publishers' privacy requirements (e.g., multiple privacy constraints that contain exactly the same ICD codes), is constructed (step 1). To avoid the unnecessary computational overhead that providing $\mathcal{P}'$ as input to an anonymization algorithm would cause, a simple pruning strategy is used (steps 2–8). First, the algorithm sorts the privacy constraints in $\mathcal{P}'$ in decreasing order based on their size and then iterates over them (steps 2 and 3). For each privacy constraint p_i in $\mathcal{P}'$, PPE deletes every privacy constraint that is a subset of p_i (steps 4–7). This results in retaining the sets of ICD codes which, when protected in $\tilde{\mathcal{D}}$, will also lead to the protection of all their subsets. After that, PPE checks if p_i is already satisfied in D, in which case p_i is removed from $\mathscr{P}'$. When all the privacy constraints in $\mathscr{P}'$ have been considered, the latter privacy policy is returned (step 13).

As an example, consider the application of PPE to *Mary*'s records in Fig. 4.1b, using $k = 5$, and the *single visit* filtering condition. First, PPE adds the privacy constraints $\{157.0, 185\}$ and $\{157.1, 157.2, 157.3\}$, which correspond to the service dates $01/02/08$ and $07/09/09$, respectively, into $\mathscr{P}'$. However, since the first privacy constraint is supported by five transactions in the dataset of Fig. 4.1b, PPE removes this constraint from $\mathscr{P}'$, and returns a privacy policy that contains only $\{157.1, 157.2, 157.3\}$.

4.3.2 Utility-Guided Anonymization of CLInical Profiles (UGACLIP)

Given $\mathscr{D}$, $\mathscr{P}$, $\mathscr{U}$, and k, the Utility-Guided Anonymization of CLInical Profiles (UGACLIP) algorithm [9] constructs an anonymized dataset $\tilde{\mathscr{D}}$ that is protected from re-identification and useful in validating GWAS. UGACLIP iterates over all privacy constraints in $\mathscr{P}$, and applies generalization and suppression until $\mathscr{P}$ is satisfied, starting with the privacy constraint that requires the least amount of information loss to be satisfied. Generalization is applied to one item i in p at a time, which is generalized in a way that incurs minimal information loss and does not violate the utility policy $\mathscr{U}$. When no item in p can be generalized without violating the specified utility policy, UGACLIP suppresses p to satisfy it, and proceeds into considering the next privacy constraint in $\mathscr{P}$. When all privacy constraints in $\mathscr{P}$ are satisfied, the algorithm returns the anonymized dataset $\tilde{\mathscr{D}}$.

The pseudocode of UGACLIP is provided in Algorithm 6. Given a dataset D, a utility policy $\mathscr{U}$, a privacy policy $\mathscr{P}$, and a parameter k, UGACLIP first initializes the anonymized database $\tilde{\mathscr{D}}$ to the original dataset $\mathscr{D}$ (step 1). Then, it selects the privacy constraint p that has the largest support in $\tilde{\mathscr{D}}$. To satisfy p, UGACLIP first checks whether the ICD codes in p can be generalized according to the utility policy $\mathscr{U}$ (step 4). If this is the case, UGACLIP selects the ICD code i from p that has the smallest support in $\tilde{\mathscr{D}}$ and finds the utility constraint u that contains i (step 5 and 6). Next, the algorithm checks if u has at least two ICD codes (this ensures that generalizing i is possible), and finds the ICD code i' from u with which i can be generalized in a way that minimizes information loss (steps 7–9). Subsequently, $\tilde{\mathscr{D}}$ is updated to reflect this generalization (step 9). In the case that u contains only one ICD code and i is supported by fewer than k transactions in $\tilde{\mathscr{D}}$, UGACLIP suppresses i and removes this ICD code from every transaction in $\tilde{D}$ that supports it (step 11 and 12). When the above steps are insufficient to satisfy the privacy constraint p, UGACLIP suppresses all items in p to satisfy it and updates $\tilde{\mathscr{D}}$ accordingly (steps 13–15). UGACLIP repeats the same process to satisfy all privacy constraints in the privacy policy $\mathscr{P}$. When all privacy constraints are satisfied, the anonymized database $\tilde{D}$ is returned as a result (step 16).

Algorithm 6 UGACLIP($\mathcal{D}, \mathcal{P}, \mathcal{U}, k$) [9]

---

    input: Dataset $\mathcal{D}$, privacy policy $\mathcal{P}$, utility policy $\mathcal{U}$, parameter k
    output: Anonymized dataset $\tilde{\mathcal{D}}$

1. $\tilde{\mathcal{D}} \leftarrow \mathcal{D}$ ▷ Initialize the anonymized database $\tilde{\mathcal{D}}$ to $\mathcal{D}$
2.   **while** privacy policy $\mathcal{P}$ is not satisfied
3. $p \leftarrow$ the privacy constraint in $\mathcal{P}$ with the maximum support in $\tilde{\mathcal{D}}$
4.   **while** p is not satisfied and items in p can be generalized without violating $\mathcal{U}$
5. $i \leftarrow$ the ICD code in p with the minimum support in $\tilde{D}$
6. $u \leftarrow$ the utility constraint from $\mathcal{U}$ that contains i
7.   **if** u contains at least two ICD codes   ▷ i can still be generalized
8.   Generalize i with another ICD code i' in u such that the $IL((i,i'))$ is minimum
9.   Update $\tilde{\mathcal{D}}$ to reflect the generalization of i and i' to (i,i')
10.   **else if** $sup(i, \tilde{\mathcal{D}}) \in (0,k)$
11.   Suppress i ▷ i is not protected and it cannot be further generalized
12.   Update $\tilde{\mathcal{D}}$ to reflect the suppression of i
13.   **if** $sup(p, \tilde{\mathcal{D}}) \in (0,k)$
14.   Suppress p
15.   Update $\tilde{\mathcal{D}}$ to reflect the suppression of p
16. **return** $\tilde{\mathcal{D}}$

As an example, consider applying UGACLIP to the data shown in Fig. 4.1a using the utility and privacy policies of Fig. 4.1c, d respectively, and $k = 5$. Since all privacy constraints have a support of 1, UGACLIP arbitrarily selects the privacy constraint $\{157.1, 157.2, 157.3\}$ and attempts to satisfy it by replacing 157.3 (the least supported ICD code in this constraint) and 157.2 with the anonymized item $(157.2, 157.3)$. This generalization minimizes information loss and satisfies the utility constraint corresponding to *Pancreatic cancer* (i.e., the number of patients suffering from this disease in the data of Fig. 4.1a is unaffected by generalization). However, the privacy constraint remains unprotected and thus $(157.2, 157.3)$ is further generalized to $(157.1, 157.2, 157.3)$. The latter generalization satisfies the utility constraint corresponding to *Pancreatic cancer*, as well as the privacy constraint $\{157.1, 157.2, 157.3\}$, since $(157.1, 157.2, 157.3)$ corresponds to at least five patients. At this point, UGACLIP proceeds by considering the next privacy constraint $\{157.9\}$. After that, UGACLIP produces the anonymized clinical profiles depicted in Fig. 4.1e.

In UGACLIP, a number of ICD codes are generalized to an anonymized item corresponding to their set, according to the specified utility policy. However, it may be impossible to protect a privacy constraint using generalization only. This occurs when, after applying all generalizations that satisfy the utility policy, a privacy constraint is supported by fewer than k transactions in $\tilde{\mathcal{D}}$. In this case, suppression is applied to remove ICD codes from the privacy constraint until this constraint is satisfied. The authors of [9] have shown that applying suppression may result in violating the utility policy, because it may reduce the number of patients associated with certain diseases, resulting in potentially invalid GWAS findings, and proposed limiting the number of allowable suppressed ICD codes via a user-specified threshold to mitigate this effect. Fortunately, GWAS tend to focus on statistically significant associations, which involve frequent ICD codes that are unlikely to be suppressed in practice for commonly-used protection levels.

4.3.3 Limitations of UGACLIP and the Clustering-Based Anonymizer (CBA)

UGACLIP is effective at preserving the specified associations between ICD codes and genomic information, but may incur high information loss when generalizing diagnosis codes that are not contained in the specified associations. In the following, we explain why this happens and discuss how the amount of information loss can be reduced. Then, Clustering-Based Anonymizer (CBA) [5], an algorithm that employs these strategies to produce data that remain useful for GWAS and general data analysis tasks, is presented.

Anonymization heuristics The first reason for which UGACLIP may heavily distort diagnosis codes that are not related to GWAS is that these codes are replaced by large anonymized items that are difficult to interpret. In fact, the IL measure, used in UGACLIP, allows creating such anonymized items, because the first term of the product in the formula of IL (see Definition 4.5) is often much smaller than the other two terms [9]. To address this issue, Gkoulalas-Divanis et al. [5] proposed the following variant of IL, which is called *Information Loss Metric (ILM)*.

Definition 4.6 (Information Loss Metric). The *Information Loss Metric (ILM)* for an anonymized item $\tilde{i_m}$ is defined as

$$ILM(\tilde{i_m}) = \frac{|\tilde{i_m}|}{M} \times w(\tilde{i_m}) \times \frac{sup(\tilde{i_m}, \tilde{\mathscr{D}})}{N}$$

where $|\tilde{i_m}|$, M, N, and w are as defined in Definition 4.5.

The Information Loss Metric differs from IL in that it penalizes large anonymized items more heavily, so that the values in all the three terms of the product are comparable. Intuitively, this allows capturing information loss more accurately.

Furthermore, UGACLIP considers generalizing a certain item i in p (i.e., the item with the minimum support in $\tilde{\mathscr{D}}$) with all items in its corresponding utility constraint to find the generalization with the lowest information loss. However, this strategy does not find the generalization with the lowest information loss, when generalizing a different item than i in p incurs lower information loss [5]. For example, consider the third privacy constraint shown in Fig. 4.1d. Since 493.01 is the least supported code in the dataset of Fig. 4.1a, UGACLIP would consider generalizing 493.01 with either 493.00 or 493.02. Assuming $w = 1$, both of these generalizations incur the same amount of information loss, and UGACLIP arbitrarily selects one of them. If $k = 2$, any of these generalizations suffices to satisfy p. However, generalizing

---

Algorithm 7 CBA($\mathscr{D}, \mathscr{P}, \mathscr{U}, k$) [5]

---

    input: Dataset $\mathscr{D}$, privacy policy $\mathscr{P}$, utility policy $\mathscr{U}$, and parameter k
    output: Anonymized dataset $\tilde{\mathscr{D}}$
1. $\tilde{\mathscr{D}} \leftarrow \mathscr{D}$
2.   Populate a priority queue PQ with all privacy constraints in $\mathscr{P}$
3.   **while** (PQ is not empty)
4.   Retrieve the top-most privacy constraint p from PQ
5.   **foreach** ($i_m \in p$)
6.   **if** (i_m is an anonymized item)
7. $\tilde{i}_m \leftarrow$ anonymized item containing the ICD codes specified by the mapping for i_m
8.   **if** ($\tilde{i}_m \in p$)
9. $p \leftarrow p \setminus i_m$
10.   **else**
11. $p \leftarrow (p \setminus i_m) \cup \tilde{i}_m$
12.   **while** ($sup(p, \tilde{\mathscr{D}}) \in (0, k)$)
13. $I \leftarrow$ find a pair $\{i_m, i_s\}$ such that i_m is contained in p, i_m and i_s are contained
                  in the same utility constraint $u \in \mathscr{U}$ and $ILM(\,(i_m, i_s)\,)$ is minimal
14.   **if**($I \neq \varnothing$)
15. $\tilde{i} \leftarrow$ anonymized item containing the ICD codes in I
16.   Update $\tilde{\mathscr{D}}$ based on $\tilde{i}$
17.   Update p by replacing i_m and/or i_s with $\tilde{i}$
18.   Store the mapping of each ICD code in $\tilde{i}$ with the set of ICD codes contained in $\tilde{i}$
19.   **else**
20.   **while**($sup(p, \tilde{\mathscr{D}}) \in (0, k)$)
21. $i_r \leftarrow$ the ICD code in p with the minimum support in $\tilde{\mathscr{D}}$
22. $p \leftarrow p \setminus i_r$
23.   Remove p from PQ
24. **return** $\tilde{\mathscr{D}}$

493.00 together with 493.02 would incur less information loss, according to both *IL* and *ILM* measures. Thus, a strategy that considers the generalization of all items in p with all items in their corresponding utility constraints and selects the best generalization in terms of information loss was proposed in [5].

Last, UGACLIP suppresses all diagnosis codes in p, when generalization alone is not sufficient to protect p. This strategy may suppress a larger than required number of diagnosis codes, particularly in the presence of strict privacy requirements. Alternatively, it is possible to suppress one diagnosis code in p at a time, until p is satisfied.

Clustering-Based Anonymizer (CBA) The pseudocode of CBA is provided in Algorithm 7. This algorithm starts by initializing a temporary dataset $\tilde{\mathscr{D}}$ to the original dataset $\mathscr{D}$ and a priority queue PQ, which stores the specified privacy constraints that have been extracted by PPE sorted w.r.t. their support in decreasing order. Then, CBA protects all privacy constraints in PQ (steps 3–14). More specifically, CBA retrieves the top-most privacy constraint p from PQ (step 4) and updates the elements of p to reflect generalizations that may have occurred in the previous iterations of CBA (step 5–11). This operation ensures that all codes in p

Fig. 4.2 Example of a research dataset

ID	Diagnoses	DNA
1	296.00 296.01 296.02	CA...T
2	295.00 295.01 295.02 295.03 295.04	TA...C
3	295.01 295.02	CT...A
4	296.00 296.02 295.02 295.03	GC...C
5	295.00 295.01 295.02 295.03	CG....A

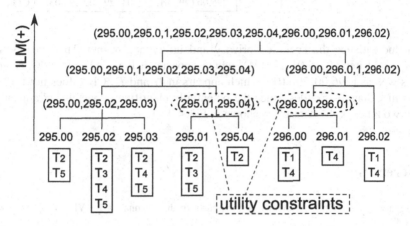

Fig. 4.3 Anonymizing the data of Fig. 4.2 using CBA

are also contained in $\tilde{\mathscr{D}}$, so that CBA can accurately determine if p is protected. To achieve this, CBA iterates over each code i_m in p and replaces it with the generalized term $\tilde{i}_m$ it is mapped to, so that p contains $\tilde{i}_m$ just once.

Then, the algorithm examines whether p needs protection, in which case it generalizes or suppresses ICD codes in it (step 12–22). Specifically, CBA utilizes the aforementioned strategy to reduce information loss caused by generalization. That is, it attempts to find a pair of codes $\{i_m, i_s\}$ that can be generalized together, according to the utility policy $\mathscr{U}$ and in a way that minimizes *ILM* (step 13). If such a pair is found, i_m and i_s are both generalized to $\tilde{i}$, the anonymized dataset $\tilde{\mathscr{D}}$ and p are updated to reflect the generalization, and the mappings between i_m and $\tilde{i}$ and between i_s and $\tilde{i}$ are stored to allow code updating (steps 16–18). If a pair $\{i_m, i_s\}$ cannot be found, then CBA iteratively suppresses codes from p, starting with the least supported code in $\tilde{\mathscr{D}}$, until p is satisfied (steps 20–22). This allows CBA to suppress no more ICD codes than what is required to protect p. After p is satisfied, it is removed from PQ (step 23), and the algorithm checks whether PQ contains another privacy constraint that must be considered. When PQ becomes empty, CBA returns the anonymized dataset $\tilde{\mathscr{D}}$ (step 24).

As an example, consider applying CBA to the data of Fig. 4.2 using a privacy policy $\mathscr{P} = \{\{295.00, \ldots, 295.04\}, \{296.0, 296.01, 296.02\}\}$, a utility policy $\mathscr{U} = \{\{295.01, 295.04\}, \{296.00, 296.01\}\}$, and $k = 2$. As can be seen in Fig. 4.3, CBA considers generalizing codes together, so that the resultant anonymization has low

Fig. 4.4 Anonymized dataset
produced by applying CBA
[5] to the dataset of Fig. 4.2

a

Diagnoses	DNA
(296.00, 296.01) 296.02	CA...T
295.00 (295.01, 295.04) 295.02 295.03	TA...C
(295.01, 295.04) 295.02	CT...A
(296.00, 296.01) 296.02 295.02 295.03	GC...C
295.00 (295.01, 295.04) 295.02 295.03	CG....A

ILM and satisfies the specified privacy and utility constraints. This creates the anonymized item $(295.01, 295.04)$, which appears in the transactions T_2, T_3 and T_5, as well as $(296.00, 296.01)$, which appears in T_1 and T_4. CBA does not further generalize diagnosis codes, since the potentially identifying codes in $\mathscr{P}$ appear at least two times in the dataset, as shown in Fig. 4.4.

References

1. Aggarwal, C.C.: On k-anonymity and the curse of dimensionality. In: VLDB, pp. 901–909 (2005)
2. Cao, J., Karras, P., Raïssi, C., Tan, K.: *rho*-uncertainty: Inference-proof transaction anonymization. PVLDB **3**(1), 1033–1044 (2010)
3. Emam, K.E., Dankar, F.K.: Protecting privacy using k-anonymity. Journal of the American Medical Informatics Association **15**(5), 627–637 (2008)
4. Fung, B.C.M., Wang, K., Chen, R., Yu, P.S.: Privacy-preserving data publishing: A survey on recent developments. ACM Comput. Surv. **42** (2010)
5. Gkoulalas-Divanis, A., Loukides, G.: PCTA: Privacy-constrained Clustering-based Transaction Data Anonymization. In: EDBT PAIS, p. 5 (2011)
6. He, Y., Naughton, J.F.: Anonymization of set-valued data via top-down, local generalization. PVLDB **2**(1), 934–945 (2009)
7. LeFevre, K., DeWitt, D., Ramakrishnan, R.: Incognito: efficient full-domain k-anonymity. In: SIGMOD, pp. 49–60 (2005)
8. Loukides, G., Denny, J., Malin, B.: The disclosure of diagnosis codes can breach research participants' privacy. Journal of the American Medical Informatics Association **17**, 322–327 (2010)
9. Loukides, G., Gkoulalas-Divanis, A., Malin, B.: Anonymization of electronic medical records for validating genome-wide association studies. Proceedings of the National Academy of Sciences **17**(107), 7898–7903 (2010)
10. Loukides, G., Gkoulalas-Divanis, A., Malin, B.: COAT: Constraint-based anonymization of transactions. KAIS **28**(2), 251–282 (2011)
11. Machanavajjhala, A., Gehrke, J., Kifer, D., Venkitasubramaniam, M.: l-diversity: Privacy beyond k-anonymity. In: ICDE, p. 24 (2006)
12. Manolio, T.A.: Collaborative genome-wide association studies of diverse diseases: programs of the nhgris office of population genomics. Pharmacogenomics **10**(2), 235–241 (2009)
13. National Institutes of Health: Policy for sharing of data obtained in NIH supported or conducted genome-wide association studies. NOT-OD-07-088. 2007.
14. Nergiz, M.E., Clifton, C.: Thoughts on k-anonymization. DKE **63**(3), 622–645 (2007)

15. Ohno-Machado, L., Vinterbo, S., Dreiseitl, S.: Effects of data anonymization by cell suppression on descriptive statistics and predictive modeling performance. Journal of American Medical Informatics Association **9**(6), 115–119 (2002)
16. Samarati, P.: Protecting respondents identities in microdata release. TKDE **13**(9), 1010–1027 (2001)
17. Sweeney, L.: k-anonymity: a model for protecting privacy. IJUFKS **10**, 557–570 (2002)
18. Terrovitis, M., Mamoulis, N., Kalnis, P.: Privacy-preserving anonymization of set-valued data. PVLDB **1**(1), 115–125 (2008)
19. Terrovitis, M., Mamoulis, N., Kalnis, P.: Local and global recoding methods for anonymizing set-valued data. VLDB J **20**(1), 83–106 (2011)
20. Xu, Y., Wang, K., Fu, A.W.C., Yu, P.S.: Anonymizing transaction databases for publication. In: KDD, pp. 767–775 (2008)

Chapter 5
Case Study on Electronic Medical Records Data

5.1 Description of Datasets and Experimental Setup

This study reports results using the *Vanderbilt Population* (*VP*) and *Vanderbilt Native Electrical Conduction* (*VNEC*) datasets [6, 7]. Recall from Chap. 3 that *VP* is derived from the de-identified version of the EMR system of the Vanderbilt University Medical Center [11], and that *VNEC* is a sample of *VP*, which is related to a GWAS on native electrical conduction within the ventricles of the heart and is expected to be released to the dbGaP repository[10]. Furthermore, a third dataset, called *VNEC Known Controls* (*VNEC_{KC}*) is also used [7]. *VNEC_{KC}* contains 1,335 records and models a scenario in which data publishers know which diagnoses can be applied as cases for other studies [1]. The characteristics of the aforementioned datasets are summarized in Table 5.1.

The following experiments, borrowed from [6,7], were performed using C++ implementations of both algorithms, and they were executed on an Intel 2.8 GHz machine with 4 GB of RAM. The default value for k was 5, and a utility policy containing ICD codes associated with GWAS-related diseases was used. For details on the construction of the utility policy, we refer the reader to [7].

5.2 The Impact of *Simple Suppression* on Preventing Data Linkage and on Data Utility

Releasing patient data intact may risk re-identification based on the attack considered in Chap. 3. However, it is natural to ask whether this attack can be prevented by releasing only ICD codes that are supported by at most s % of the records of the population dataset. This strategy is termed *simple suppression* and effectively assumes that each patient is represented by a single record with one diagnosis code. Simple suppression is similar in principle to the strategy proposed by Vinterbo et al. [13]. Figure 5.2b, which is borrowed from [6], investigates the

Table 5.1 Description of the datasets used

Dataset	N	$|\mathscr{I}|$	Max. number of ICD codes per record	Avg. number of ICD codes per record
VP	1,174,793	13,538	370	3
$VNEC$	2,762	5,830	25	3.1
$VNEC_{KC}$	1,335	305	3.1	5.0

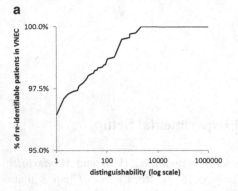
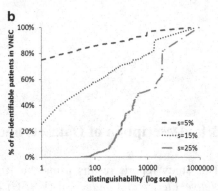

Fig. 5.1 Percentage of patient records in $VNEC$ that are vulnerable to re-identification when (**a**) data are released in their original form, and (**b**) when ICD codes in $VNEC$, which are supported by at most $s\%$ of records in VP, are suppressed [6]

impact of simple suppression on preventing the aforementioned attack, using the distinguishability measure (see Sect. 3.3). This figure suggests that approximately 75 and 26 % of patient records in $VNEC$ are vulnerable to the attack when the ICD codes are supported by no more than 5 and 15 % of the records in VP, respectively. On the contrary, to prevent re-identification, all ICD codes supported by no more than 25 % of the records in VP had to be suppressed.

While applying simple suppression using $s = 25\%$ can prevent the attack, it is important to consider how useful the suppressed data are. To capture data utility, the measures of Sect. 3.4 are employed, and results, which are borrowed from [6], are presented.

In the first set of results, dataset-level measures are considered. Table 5.2a reports the percentage of retained disease information in $VNEC$ after applying simple suppression with an s value in $\{5, 15, 25\%\}$. Observe that the percent of five-digit ICD codes, three-digit ICD codes and ICD sections retained was at most 2, 7 and 25.4 % respectively. These results indicate that simple suppression may lead to high information loss. Moreover, setting s to 25 %, the lowest value that results in a distinguishability of more than 1, results in retaining very little information. Specifically, only 0.1, 0.7, and 3.2 % of five-digit ICD codes, three-digit ICD codes and ICD sections, respectively, are retained. The disease information retained at different aggregation levels is illustrated in Table 5.2b. This information may be too general to be of assistance for GWAS, because large categories of diagnoses have been suppressed (see [6] for details).

Table 5.2 (a) Percentage of retained disease information after applying simple suppression with varying s, and (b) disease information retained after applying simple suppression with varying s [6]

(a)

$s\%$	5-digit (%)	3-digit (%)	Sections (%)
5	1.8	6.7	25.4
15	0.3	1.5	7.9
25	0.1	0.7	3.2

(b)

5-digit	3-digit	Sections
401.1	401	Hypertensive
Benign essential hypertension	Essential hypertension	disease
780.79	780	Rheumatism excluding
Other malaise and fatigue	Other soft tissue	the back
729.5	729	Rheumatism excluding
Pain in limb	Other disorders of soft tissue	the back
789.0	789	Symptoms
Abdominal pain	Other abdomen/pelvis syptoms	
786.65	786	Symptoms
Chest pain	Respir. system and other chest symptoms	

In the second set of results, data utility is captured at a record level, using the *SL* and *RSL* measures (see Sect. 3.4). The *SL* scores for simple suppression with s set to 5, 15, and 25 % are reported in Fig. 5.2a. As can be observed, increasing the level of suppression applied, results in less data utility, due to the trade-off between utility and privacy [8]. Nevertheless, 14 ICD codes were suppressed from more than 52 % of the transactions in all tested s values. The *RSL* scores for the same suppression levels are shown in Fig. 5.2b. Observe that the percent of suppressed ICD codes of the transactions was more than 60 % in all tested suppression levels, while all of the ICD codes of more than 18 % of the transactions had to be suppressed at a suppression level of 25 %, which prevents re-identification. These results verify that suppression may heavily distort data, reducing data utility significantly.

5.3 Utility of Anonymized Diagnosis Codes

In this section, the effectiveness of the UGACLIP and CBA algorithms at preserving data utility is evaluated in terms of their ability to construct useful anonymizations for validating GWAS, as well as to help studies focusing on clinical case counts. These algorithms are compared against *ACLIP* (Anonymization of CLInical Profiles), a variant of UGACLIP, which was proposed in [7]. ACLIP uses the same privacy policy as UGACLIP, but it does not take the utility policy into account. Rather, ACLIP attempts to minimize information loss. In this sense, ACLIP is similar to the premise of the anonymization approaches proposed in [4, 12, 14].

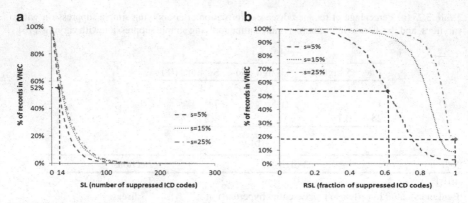

Fig. 5.2 Data utility after applying simple suppression, as it is captured by (**a**) *SL*, and (**b**) *RSL* [6]

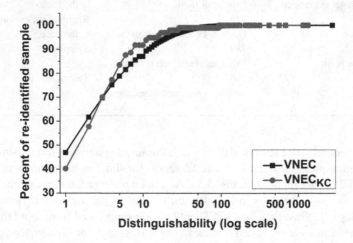

Fig. 5.3 Re-identification risk (shown as a cumulative distribution function) of clinical profiles [7]

Note that both the *VNEC* and *VNEC$_{KC}$* datasets are susceptible to the attack described in Chap. 4, in which an attacker knows that a patient's record is contained in the published data. This is evident in Fig. 5.3, which reports the *distinguishability* (i.e., the number of records in the published dataset that share a set of potentially linkable ICD code) for the *single-visit* filtering condition and is borrowed from [7]. Notice, at least 40 % of the records of each dataset are uniquely identifiable.

5.3.1 Supporting GWAS Validation

In this section, the effectiveness of UGACLIP at generating anonymizations that allow GWAS validation is considered. First, the number of utility constraints the anonymized clinical profiles satisfy is reported, for the *VNEC* dataset, in Fig. 5.4a.

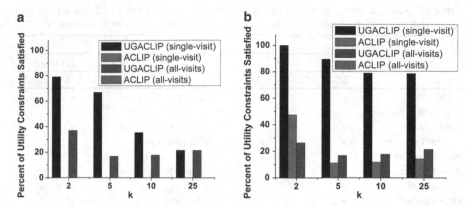

Fig. 5.4 Utility constraint satisfaction at various levels of protection for: (**a**) *VNEC*, and (**b**) $VNEC_{KC}$ [6]

Note that the anonymizations generated by UGACLIP with $k = 5$, as is often in applications [2], satisfied more than 66 % of the specified utility constraints for the single visit case. As expected, the number of satisfied utility constraints dropped for the all visits case. However, UGACLIP still satisfied at least 16.7 % of the utility constraints for all k values. This is in contrast to ACLIP, which failed to construct a useful result for GWAS (no utility constraints were satisfied in any case). The result of applying UGACLIP and ACLIP to the $VNEC_{KC}$ dataset, reported in Fig. 5.4b, is quantitatively similar to that of Fig. 5.4a. These results suggest that UGACLIP is effective in anonymizing data guided by a utility policy. Interestingly, applying both methods to $VNEC_{KC}$ resulted in an increased number of satisfied utility constraints. This is because restricting clinical profiles to diseases related to GWAS makes $VNEC_{KC}$ less sparse than $VNEC$, which increases the chance of grouping ICD codes in a way that satisfies utility constraints.

Furthermore, it was examined which of the utility constraints are satisfied by the anonymized data. Table 5.3a depicts the results for the single visit case, for $k = 2$. Notice that the anonymized data produced by UGACLIP validate GWAS-related associations for most of the diseases (79 and 100 % for *VNEC* and *VNEC*, respectively). On the contrary, ACLIP generated data that fail to satisfy any of the utility constraints and, thus, cannot be used in validating GWAS for the selected diseases. The corresponding results for the all-visits case are shown in Table 5.3b. Note that UGACLIP still managed to satisfy 28 and 39 % of the utility constraints in the case of *VNEC* and $VNEC_{KC}$, respectively, while ACLIP satisfied none of these constraints, in any of these cases. This setting clearly shows that UGACLIP can produce data that helps GWAS validation, even when data publishers have strict privacy requirements.

Table 5.4a illustrates which of the utility constraints are satisfied in the anonymized datasets produced by UGACLIP and CBA, for $k = 5$ and in the single-visit case. As can be seen from this table, the anonymizations generated by CBA

Table 5.3 Satisfied utility constraints for UGACLIP and ACLIP when $k = 2$ and for (**a**) the single-visit case, and (**b**) the all-visits case (✓ denotes that a utility constraint is satisfied) [7]

(a)

Disease	VNEC		VNEC$_{KC}$		Disease	VNEC		VNEC$_{KC}$	
	UGA	ACL	UGA	ACL		UGA	ACL	UGA	ACL
Asthma	✓		✓	✓	Lung cancer	✓		✓	
Attention deficit with					Major depressive dis.			✓	
hyperactivity	✓		✓		Pancreatic cancer	✓		✓	✓
Bipolar I disorder	✓		✓	✓	Platelet phenotypes			✓	
Bladder cancer	✓		✓	✓	Pre-term birth	✓		✓	✓
Breast cancer	✓		✓		Prostate cancer	✓		✓	
Coronary disease	✓		✓	✓	Psoriasis	✓		✓	✓
Dental caries	✓		✓		Renal cancer	✓		✓	
Diabetes mellitus type-1	✓		✓	✓	Schizophrenia			✓	
Diabetes mellitus type-2	✓		✓	✓	Sickle-cell disease			✓	

(b)

Disease	VNEC		VNEC$_{KC}$		Disease	VNEC		VNEC$_{KC}$	
	UGA	ACL	UGA	ACL		UGA	ACL	UGA	ACL
Asthma					Lung cancer	✓		✓	
Attention deficit with					Pancreatic cancer	✓		✓	
hyperactivity					Platelet phenotypes				
Bipolar I disorder			✓		Pre-term birth				
Bladder cancer					Prostate cancer	✓		✓	
Breast cancer			✓		Psoriasis				
Coronary disease					Renal cancer				
Dental caries					Schizophrenia				
Diabetes mellitus type-1	✓		✓		Sickle-cell disease				
Diabetes mellitus type-2	✓		✓						

satisfied 22.2 and 5.5 % more utility constraints than those created by UGACLIP for $VNEC$ and $VNEC_{KC}$, respectively. The result of the same experiment, but with $k = 10$, is reported in Table 5.4b. This experiment shows that CBA outperformed UGACLIP by a margin of 29.4 % for both datasets. This confirms the analysis of Sect. 4.3.3 which showed that selecting a fixed ICD code for generalization, as UGACLIP does, incurs a large amount of information loss, particularly when k is large.

5.3.2   Supporting Clinical Case Count Studies

The effectiveness of UGACLIP and CBA in producing data that assist clinical case count studies, which are beyond GWAS-specific validation, is also important to consider. This is because it may be difficult for data publishers to a priori predict all possible uses of GWAS data. Specifically, it is assumed that data recipients issue

Table 5.4 Satisfied utility constraints for UGACLIP and CBA for the single-visit case when (a) $k = 5$, and (b) $k = 10$ (✓ denotes that a utility constraint is satisfied) [3]

Disease	VNEC UGA	VNEC CBA	VNEC_KC UGA	VNEC_KC CBA	Disease	VNEC UGA	VNEC CBA	VNEC_KC UGA	VNEC_KC CBA
Asthma	✓	✓	✓	✓	Lung cancer	✓	✓	✓	✓
Attention deficit with hyperactivity	✓		✓		Pancreatic cancer	✓	✓	✓	✓
Bipolar I disorder		✓		✓	Platelet phenotypes	✓		✓	
Bladder cancer	✓		✓		Pre-term birth	✓	✓	✓	✓
Breast cancer	✓	✓	✓	✓	Prostate cancer	✓	✓	✓	✓
Coronary disease		✓		✓	Psoriasis	✓		✓	✓
Dental caries	✓	✓	✓	✓	Renal cancer	✓		✓	✓
Diabetes mellitus type-1	✓	✓	✓		Schizophrenia	✓		✓	✓
Diabetes mellitus type-2	✓	✓	✓		Sickle-cell disease	✓		✓	✓

(a)

Disease	VNEC UGA	VNEC CBA	VNEC_KC UGA	VNEC_KC CBA	Disease	VNEC UGA	VNEC CBA	VNEC_KC UGA	VNEC_KC CBA
Asthma	✓	✓	✓	✓	Diabetes mellitus type-2	✓	✓	✓	
Attention deficit with hyperactivity					Lung cancer			✓	
Bipolar I disorder	✓		✓	✓	Pancreatic cancer				
Bladder cancer	✓		✓		Platelet phenotypes	✓		✓	
Breast cancer		✓	✓	✓	Pre-term birth	✓		✓	✓
Coronary disease	✓	✓	✓	✓	Prostate cancer	✓		✓	✓
Dental caries	✓	✓	✓	✓	Psoriasis	✓		✓	✓
Diabetes mellitus type-1	✓	✓	✓		Renal cancer	✓		✓	✓
					Schizophrenia	✓		✓	✓

(b)

```
Q: SELECT COUNT(*)
   FROM dataset
   WHERE ICD_1 ∈ dataset and ICD_2 ∈ dataset and ... and ICD_q ∈ dataset
```

Fig. 5.5 Example of a query that requires counting the number of patients diagnosed with a certain set of ICD codes

queries to learn the number of patient records harboring a set of ICD codes that are supported by at least 10 % of the transactions. This task is crucial in medical data mining applications [14], as well as in epidemiology, where combinations of diagnoses form syndromes [9]. However, anonymized data may not allow such queries to be answered accurately, because an anonymized item can be interpreted as any of the non-empty subsets of ICD codes it contains. Utility is evaluated using *Relative Error* (*RE*) [5], which reflects the number of records that are incorrectly retrieved in the answer to a query when issued against anonymized data. To see how *RE* can be computed, consider the following SQL-style query Q, which requires counting the number of patients diagnosed with a certain set of ICD codes.

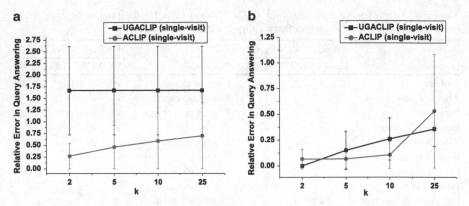

Fig. 5.6 Relative Error (*RE*) vs. *k* for the single visit case and for (**a**) *VNEC*, and (**b**) *VNEC_KC* (points correspond to the mean of *RE* scores and error bars are of 1 SD) [7]

Assume that $a(Q)$ is the answer of applying Q to the original dataset, which can be obtained by counting the number of records in this dataset that contain a certain set of ICD codes. When the same query Q is applied on the anonymized version of the dataset, an estimated answer $e(Q)$ is obtained, since the anonymized items may not allow distinguishing the actual ICD codes of a patient. To compute $e(Q)$, we first need to compute the probability a patient is diagnosed with the requested ICD code(s). The latter probability can be computed as $\prod_{r=1}^{q} p(i_r)$, where $p(i_r)$ is the probability of mapping an ICD code i_r in query Q to an anonymized item $\tilde{i}_m$, assuming that $\tilde{i}_m$ can include any possible subset of the ICD codes mapped to it with equal probability, and that there exist no correlations among the anonymized items. The estimated answer $e(Q)$ is then derived by summing the corresponding probabilities across the records of the anonymized dataset. Once $a(Q)$ and $e(Q)$ are known, the *Relative Error* (RE) for Q is given by $RE(Q) = |a(Q) - e(Q)|/a(Q)$. Intuitively, the lower the *RE* score for a workload of queries, the higher the quality of the anonymization method as it can more accurately compute from the anonymized clinical profiles the number of patients' records that correctly answer the query.

In the following experiments, borrowed from [3, 7], the mean and/or standard deviation of the *RE* scores for a workload of queries is measured. The results for the single visit case and for the *VNEC* dataset are reported in Fig. 5.6. Observe that ACLIP resulted in a relatively small error, less than 0.75 on average, for all tested values of *k*, outperforming UGACLIP. This is because the majority of the combinations of ICD codes contained in the queries did not correspond to diseases used as control variables in GWAS, whose distribution UGACLIP was configured to preserve. Thus, as expected, UGACLIP generalized other ICD codes slightly more to preserve the distribution of these diseases. Yet, the *RE* scores for ACLIP and UGACLIP were approximately within one standard deviation of each other, for all *k* values. This suggests that UGACLIP is capable of producing anonymizations that support both GWAS and studies focusing on clinical case counts. Similar results were obtained for *VNEC_KC*, which are shown in Fig. 5.6b.

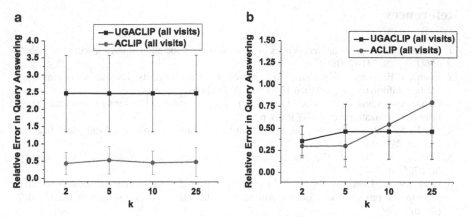

Fig. 5.7 Relative Error (*RE*) vs. *k* for the all-visits case and for (**a**) *VNEC*, and (**b**) *VNEC_{KC}* [7]

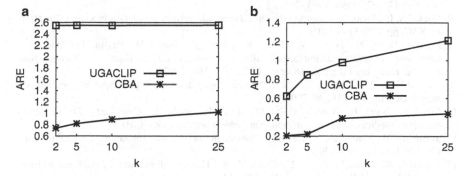

Fig. 5.8 Mean of Relative Error (*ARE*) vs. *k* for the single-visits case and for (**a**) *VNEC*, and (**b**) *VNEC_{KC}* [3]

The all-visits case was also considered. Figure 5.7a, b show the results for *VNEC* and *VNEC_{KC}*, respectively. As can be seen, the *RE* scores for both UGACLIP and ACLIP were relatively small, but larger of those in the single-visit case, due to the utility/privacy trade-off. Again, the performance of UGACLIP was comparable to, or even better than, that of ACLIP. This is explained by the fact that the queried combinations of ICD codes were contained in the utility policy used in UGACLIP, and thus were not substantially distorted.

Last, a comparison of UGACLIP to CBA for the single-visit case and for the same query workloads as in the previous experiment, is presented. Figure 5.8a, b illustrate the mean of *RE* scores for *VNEC* and *VNEC_{KC}* respectively. Observe that CBA significantly outperformed UGACLIP, as it generated anonymizations that permit at least 2.5 times more accurate querying answering. This shows the effectiveness of CBA in minimizing information loss, which is attributed to the *ILM* measure and the anonymization heuristics it employs.

References

1. Donnelly, P.: Progress and challenges in genome-wide association studies in humans. Nature **456**(11), 728–731 (2008)
2. Emam, K.E., Dankar, F.K.: Protecting privacy using k-anonymity. Journal of the American Medical Informatics Association **15**(5), 627–637 (2008)
3. Gkoulalas-Divanis, A., Loukides, G.: PCTA: Privacy-constrained Clustering-based Transaction Data Anonymization. In: EDBT PAIS, p. 5 (2011)
4. He, Y., Naughton, J.F.: Anonymization of set-valued data via top-down, local generalization. PVLDB **2**(1), 934–945 (2009)
5. LeFevre, K., DeWitt, D., Ramakrishnan, R.: Mondrian multidimensional k-anonymity. In: ICDE, p. 25 (2006)
6. Loukides, G., Denny, J., Malin, B.: The disclosure of diagnosis codes can breach research participants' privacy. Journal of the American Medical Informatics Association **17**, 322–327 (2010)
7. Loukides, G., Gkoulalas-Divanis, A., Malin, B.: Anonymization of electronic medical records for validating genome-wide association studies. Proceedings of the National Academy of Sciences **17**(107), 7898–7903 (2010)
8. Loukides, G., Shao, J.: Capturing data usefulness and privacy protection in k-anonymisation. In: SAC, pp. 370–374 (2007)
9. Marsden-Haug, N., Foster, V., Gould, P., Elbert, E., Wang, H., Pavlin, J.: Code-based syndromic surveillance for influenzalike illness by international classification of diseases, ninth revision. Emerging Infectious Diseases **13**(2), 207–216 (2007)
10. MD, M.D.M., M, M.F., Jin, Y., et al.: The ncbi dbgap database of genotypes and phenotypes. Nature Genetics **39**, 1181–6 (2007)
11. Stead, W., Bates, R., Byrd, J., Giuse, D., Miller, R., Shultz, E.: Case study: The vanderbilt university medical center information management architecture (2003)
12. Terrovitis, M., Mamoulis, N., Kalnis, P.: Privacy-preserving anonymization of set-valued data. PVLDB **1**(1), 115–125 (2008)
13. Vinterbo, S., Ohno-Machado, L., Dreiseitl, S.: Hiding information by cell suppression. In: AMIA Annual Symposium, pp. 223–228 (2001)
14. Xu, Y., Wang, K., Fu, A.W.C., Yu, P.S.: Anonymizing transaction databases for publication. In: KDD, pp. 767–775 (2008)

Chapter 6
Conclusions and Open Research Challenges

In this book, we have explained why EMR data need to be disseminated in a way that prevents patient re-identification. We have provided an overview of data sharing policies and regulations, which serve as a first line of defence but are unable to provide computational privacy guarantees, and then reviewed several anonymization approaches that can be used to prevent this threat. Specifically, we have surveyed anonymization principles and algorithms for demographics and diagnosis codes, which are high replicable, available, and distinguishable, and thus may lead to patient re-identification. Anonymity threats and methods for publishing patient information, contained in genomic data, have also been discussed.

Following that, we focused on re-identification attacks that are based on diagnosis codes. These attacks may result in associating patients with their genomic information and cannot be thwarted by de-identification and naive suppression-based strategies. Motivated by this observation, we presented an approach for producing anonymized data that help GWAS validation. This approach automatically extracts potentially identifying diagnosis codes and generalizes them, using either the UGACLIP or the CBA algorithm. Generalization is performed in a way that prevents an attacker from linking a genomic sequence to a small number of patients, while the associations between genomic sequences and specific sets of clinical features, which correspond to GWAS-related diseases, are preserved. In addition, the feasibility of these attacks was shown in experiments with data derived from the EMR system of the Vanderbilt University Medical Center. These experiments also verified that the aforementioned anonymization approach can eliminate the threat of individual re-identification, while producing data that supports GWAS validation and clinical case analysis tasks.

The book investigated a typical medical data sharing setting, in which a data publisher needs to disseminate EMR data in a way that forestalls re-identification [5, 6, 18, 24, 27]. However, there are several open research challenges that warrant further research. These challenges include an investigation of additional threats

A. Gkoulalas-Divanis and G. Loukides, *Anonymization of Electronic Medical Records to Support Clinical Analysis*, SpringerBriefs in Electrical and Computer Engineering, DOI 10.1007/978-1-4614-5668-1_6, © The Author(s) 2013

to patient privacy and the development of privacy technologies for alternative data publishing scenarios. We discuss these two challenges in Sects. 6.1 and 6.2, respectively.

6.1 Threats Beyond Patient Re-identification

Re-identification is arguably the main threat in patient-specific data publishing. However, the increasing availability of EMR data and tools to process them [11] may pose additional threats to patient privacy.

First, patient-specific data containing diagnosis codes may be susceptible to sensitive information disclosure attacks, in which an individual is associated with one or more sensitive items, as discussed in Chap. 2. To publish these data, it is important to develop approaches that are able to: (1) prevent both identity and sensitive information disclosure, which is essential to comply with existing data sharing policies and regulations, (2) deal with detailed privacy requirements, which data publishers often have, and (3) guarantee that anonymized data remain useful for biomedical tasks, including, but not limited to, GWAS. One way to achieve this is to generalize data in a way that satisfies the utility constraints, while enforcing the rule-based privacy model [16], which enables the specification of detailed privacy requirements. This calls for new anonymization models and algorithms and is a promising avenue for future work.

Second, most of the privacy models considered so far [13, 15, 17, 24, 28] assume that an attacker knows whether or not an individual's record is contained in the published dataset. However, healthcare providers often disseminate a sample that contains the records of patients diagnosed with certain diseases and is derived from a larger patient population. When these diseases are sensitive, the inference that a patient's record is contained in the sample may breach privacy. Nergiz et al. [21, 22] have studied this attack, which is termed *membership disclosure*, and noted that it may occur even when data are protected from identity and/or sensitive disclosure. In addition, they proposed anonymization algorithms for preventing membership disclosure in relational data publishing. However, such attacks may also occur in transaction data publishing (e.g., when the diagnosis codes and DNA sequences of patients with schizophrenia are released for the purposes of a GWAS on this disease) and preventing them is important.

Third, patient data that are released for mining tasks may be susceptible to *aggregate disclosure* [4]. This involves attackers who are able to infer knowledge patterns that violate patient privacy. Consider, for example, that an insurance company obtains transaction data from a hospital and applies classification to discover that patients over 40 living in an area with zipcode 33100 have a very high hospitalization cost. Based on this knowledge, the insurance company may decide to offer more expensive coverage to these patients. Thus, sensitive knowledge patterns need to be identified prior to data publishing and be hidden, so that they cannot be mined from the published data. Works that suppress selected items from sensitive knowledge patterns to hide association rules [8,9,19,23,25,26,29,32], classification rules [1,3,20], or frequent sequences [7] have been proposed. The characteristics of medical datasets, however, pose new challenges to traditional data mining methods [2] that require specialized mining approaches [12,33]. Thus, developing algorithms for hiding sensitive knowledge patterns, so that they cannot be mined by medical data mining methods, needs to be considered.

6.2 Complex Data Sharing Scenarios

The focus of this book was on a common scenario involving a single healthcare provider, who seeks to anonymize a dataset containing EMR data and then publish it to multiple other parties. In the following, we discuss two alternative scenarios that together cover a wide range of applications that benefit from EMR data publishing.

The first scenario is related to publishing heterogeneous datasets that contain information of different types (e.g., records containing both demographics and diagnosis codes), which is increasingly needed to support medical analysis tasks. Preserving privacy in heterogeneous data publishing is non-trivial, because it is expected that an attacker will have knowledge about multiple types of attributes (e.g., about a patients' age and diagnosis codes). This implies that simply splitting records horizontally, so that each part contains a different type of data, and anonymizing each part separately, using existing methods, will not preserve privacy, and new methods are required.

The last scenario we consider involves multiple healthcare providers and data recipients (e.g., medical scientists or professionals), who are using a common biorepository. Healthcare providers contribute possibly different part of a patient's EMR to the repository, based on the interaction of the patient with them, whereas data recipients pose queries to the repository. This setting presents two challenges that need to be overcome [14]. First, data contributed by different healthcare providers need to be integrated without revealing patients' identity, which is difficult to be performed in an effective and efficient way, using existing methods [10, 30]. Second, the queries answers derived from integrated data must be anonymized to guard against patient re-identification in accordance with data privacy and utility requirements. This can result in better data utility in comparison to existing approaches that anonymize all data at once [31] and answer queries using a priori anonymized parts on the transformed dataset. However, achieving privacy in this scenario is non-trivial, because an attacker may stitch together parts that are anonymized on-the-fly to re-identify patients, even when each of these views prevents re-identification when examined independently of the others.

References

1. Chen, K., Liu, L.: Privacy preserving data classification with rotation perturbation. In: ICDM, pp. 589–592 (2005)
2. Cios, K.J., Moore, G.W.: Uniqueness of medical data mining. Artificial Intelligence in Medicine **26**(1–2), 1–24 (2002)
3. Clifton, C.: Using sample size to limit exposure to data mining. J. of Computer Security **8**(4), 281–307 (2000)
4. Das, G., Zhang, N.: Privacy risks in health databases from aggregate disclosure. In: PETRA, pp. 1–4 (2009)
5. Emam, K.E.: Methods for the de-identification of electronic health records for genomic research. Genome Medicine **3**(4), 25 (2011)
6. Fienberg, S.E., Slavkovic, A., Uhler, C.: Privacy preserving gwas data sharing. In: IEEE ICDM Worksops, pp. 628–635 (2011)
7. Gkoulalas-Divanis, A., Loukides, G.: Revisiting sequential pattern hiding to enhance utility. In: KDD, pp. 1316–1324 (2011)
8. Gkoulalas-Divanis, A., Verykios, V.S.: Exact knowledge hiding through database extension. TKDE **21**(5), 699–713 (2009)
9. Gkoulalas-Divanis, A., Verykios, V.S.: Hiding sensitive knowledge without side effects. KAIS **20**(3), 263–299 (2009)
10. Hall, R., Fienberg, S.E.: Privacy-preserving record linkage. In: Privacy in Statistical Databases, pp. 269–283 (2010)
11. Hristidis, V.: Information Discovery on Electronic Health Records. Data Mining and Knowledge Discovery. Chapman and Hall/CRC (2009)
12. Jin, H., Chen, J., He, H., G.Williams, Kelman, C., OKeefe, C.: Mining unexpected temporal associations: Applications in detecting adverse drug reactions. IEEE TITB **12**(4), 488500 (2008)
13. Li, N., Li, T., Venkatasubramanian, S.: t-closeness: Privacy beyond k-anonymity and l-diversity. In: ICDE, pp. 106–115 (2007)
14. Loukides, G., Gkoulalas-Divanis, A., Malin, B.: An integrative framework for anonymizing clinical and genomic data. In: C. Plant (ed.) Database technology for life sciences and medicine, pp. 65–89. World scientific (2010)
15. Loukides, G., Gkoulalas-Divanis, A., Malin, B.: COAT: Constraint-based anonymization of transactions. KAIS **28**(2), 251–282 (2011)
16. Loukides, G., Gkoulalas-Divanis, A., Shao, J.: Anonymizing transaction data to eliminate sensitive inferences. In: DEXA, pp. 400–415 (2010)
17. Machanavajjhala, A., Gehrke, J., Kifer, D., Venkitasubramaniam, M.: l-diversity: Privacy beyond k-anonymity. In: ICDE, p. 24 (2006)
18. Malin, B., Loukides, G., Benitez, K., Clayton, E.: Identifiability in biobanks: models, measures, and mitigation strategies. Human Genetics **130**(3), 383–392 (2011)
19. Moustakides, G.V., Verykios, V.S.: A max-min approach for hiding frequent itemsets. ICDM Workshops pp. 502–506 (2006)
20. Natwichai, J., Li, X., Orlowska, M.: Hiding classification rules for data sharing with privacy preservation. In: DAWAK, pp. 468–467 (2005)
21. Nergiz, M.E., Atzori, M., Clifton, C.: Hiding the presence of individuals from shared databases. In: SIGMOD '07, pp. 665–676 (2007)
22. Nergiz, M.E., Clifton, C.W.: d-presence without complete world knowledge. TKDE **22**(6), 868–883 (2010)
23. Oliveira, S.R.M., Zaïane, O.R.: Protecting sensitive knowledge by data sanitization. In: ICDM, pp. 613–616 (2003)
24. Samarati, P.: Protecting respondents identities in microdata release. TKDE **13**(9), 1010–1027 (2001)

25. Saygin, Y., Verykios, V., Clifton, C.: Using unknowns to prevent discovery of association rules. SIGMOD Record **30**(4), 45–54 (2001)
26. Sun, X., Yu, P.S.: A border-based approach for hiding sensitive frequent itemsets. 5th IEEE International Conference on Data Mining p. 8 (2005)
27. Sweeney, L.: k-anonymity: a model for protecting privacy. IJUFKS **10**, 557–570 (2002)
28. Terrovitis, M., Mamoulis, N., Kalnis, P.: Privacy-preserving anonymization of set-valued data. PVLDB **1**(1), 115–125 (2008)
29. Verykios, V.S., Gkoulalas-Divanis, A.: A Survey of Association Rule Hiding Methods for Privacy, chap. 11, pp. 267–289. Privacy Preserving Data Mining: Models and Algorithms. Springer (2008)
30. Winkler, W.: Record linkage and bayesian networks. In: Section on Survey Research Methods, American Statistical Association (2002)
31. Xiao, X., Tao, Y.: M-invariance: towards privacy preserving re-publication of dynamic datasets. In: SIGMOD, pp. 689–700 (2007)
32. Y. Sung, Y., Liu, Y., Xiong, H., Ng, A.: Privacy preservation for data cubes. Knowledge Information Systems **9**(1), 38–61 (2006)
33. Yanqing, J., Hao, Y., Dews, P., Mansour, A., Tran, J., Miller, R., Massanari, R.: A potential causal association mining algorithm for screening adverse drug reactions in postmarketing surveillance. IEEE TITB **15**(3), 428 –437 (2011)

Index

A

aggregate disclosure, 66
all-visits, 59, 63
anonymization, 5
  algorithms
    apriori algorithm, 22
    CBA algorithm, 49
    greedy algorithm, 23, 24
    LRA-VPA algorithms, 23
    optimization objectives, 13
    partition algorithm, 19–21
    search strategies, 12
    SupressControl algorithm, 25
    UGACLIP algorithm, 47
    value recording models, 13
  principles, 9
    (h, k, p)-coherence, 17, 18
    ρ-uncertainty, 18
    (a,k)-anonymity, 11
    k-anonymity, 9, 10
    l-diversity, 11
    p-sensitive-k-anonymity, 11
    t-closeness, 11
    k^m-anonymity, 16
    complete k-anonymity, 16
    personalized privacy, 12
    privacy skyline, 11
    recursive (c,l)-diversity, 11
    worst group protection, 12
anonymized item, 43

C

case count studies, 60

D

data utility, *see* utility
dbGaP database, 2, 4, 27, 31

de-identification, 3
differential privacy, 5, 27
discharge records, 32
distinguishability, 33–35
DNA, 26, 32

E

Electronic Medical Record systems, 1, 32, 33, 39, 46
  adoption, 2
  anonymity, 2
  secrecy, 2
  security, 2
eMERGE network, 2

G

generalization
  models, 14, 18
genome-wide association study, 26, 27, 31, 49, 57, 58
genomic sequence, 26

H

heterogeneous datasets, 67
HIPAA, 2, 31
  Expert determination, 2, 4
  Safe harbor, 2
Homer's attack, 26, 27
hospital discharge records, *see* discharge records

I

ICD-9 codes, 15, 31, 32
  hierarchy, 36

A. Gkoulalas-Divanis and G. Loukides, *Anonymization of Electronic Medical Records to Support Clinical Analysis*, SpringerBriefs in Electrical and Computer Engineering, DOI 10.1007/978-1-4614-5668-1, © The Author(s) 2013

identity disclosure, *see* re-identification
information loss measure, 45, 49

J
journalist scenario, 32

M
membership disclosure, 66
microaggregation, 13
minor allele frequencies, 26
mole, 23

N
National Institutes of Health, 2, 31
non-perturbative methods, 5, 9

P
perturbative methods, 5, 9
privacy policy, 40, 42
    extraction, 45, 46
    satisfiability, 42
privacy requirements, 40

Q
quasi-identifier, 9

R
range disclosure, 12
re-identification, 3, 9
    attacks, 3, 39, 40

challenges, 4, 5, 39
risk, 4, 9, 33, 34
    distinguisability, 14
    replication, 14
    resource availability, 14
relative error, 61
relative size loss, 37

S
semantic disclosure, 11
sensitive association rule, 25
sensitive attributes, 9, 10
sensitive disclosure, *see* sensitive
        attributes
single nucleotide polymorphism, 26, 27
single visit, 58, 62
size loss, 37
suppression, 13, 55

T
transaction dataset, 15, 16
    itemset, 15
    support, 16

U
utility, 5, 36, 57
    policy, 40, 42
        satisfiability, 42
    utility requirements, 40

V
value disclosure, 10